The Intelligent Patient Guide To

Osteoporosis

Dr. Roger A.L. Sutton
Dr. Robert G. Josse

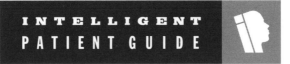

INTELLIGENT
PATIENT GUIDE

First edition, Vancouver, 2009

Distributed by
Gordon Soules Book Publishers Ltd.
1359 Ambleside Lane,
West Vancouver, BC, Canada V7T 2Y9
E-mail: books@gordonsoules.com
Web site: http://www.gordonsoules.com
(604) 922 6588 Fax: (604) 688 5442

While the authors have made every effort to ensure that the material contained herein is accurate at time of publication, new discoveries or changes in treatment practices may ultimately invalidate some of the information presented here.

Intelligent Patient Guide Ltd.
Suite 30, 3195 Granville Street
Vancouver, British Columbia V6H 3K2
Canada
e-mail: info@ipguide.com
fax: 604-876-9334

Library and Archives Canada Cataloguing in Publication

Sutton, Roger A. L
    The intelligent patient guide to osteoporosis / Roger A. L. Sutton,
Robert G. Josse ; edited by Cheryl Edwards ; illustrated by Vicky L. Earle.

(Intelligent patient guide)
Includes index.
ISBN 978-0-9811599-0-4

    1. Osteoporosis—Popular works. I. Josse, Robert G., 1946-
II. Edwards, Cheryl, 1950- III. Earle, Vicky. IV. Title.
V. Series: Intelligent patient guide

RC931.O73S89 2009   616.7'16   C2008-907914-0

Praise for *The Intelligent Patient Guide to Osteoporisis*

*Exercise, take enough calcium and vitamin D, and read this book!
Drs. Sutton and Josse give your skeleton the respect it deserves by
pouring a combined sixty years of osteoporosis management into a
guide that dramatically raises the bar for patient education materials.
Absolutely everything you need to know to take an active part in your
treatment, including a much needed wake-up call for all those men who
thought osteoporosis was just an older woman's disease. My patients
love these Intelligent Patient Guides. They come equipped with all the
right questions, they expect answers, and they get them.*

— S. Larry Goldenberg, OBC MD FRCSC
Professor and Head, Department of Urologic Sciences
University of British Columbia
Director of Men's Health Initiative

*This is a lovely book. It is written by two eminent investigators who
clearly are passionate and committed to their field of research and have
produced a book that has everything. It is easily accessible to the reader.
In some ways, it is so comprehensive that doctors will benefit from its
clear and insightful yet measured evaluation of the problem of
osteoporosis and how it can be detected, prevented and treated.*

— Ego Seeman
Professor of Medicine
Austin Health The University of Melbourne
Melbourne, Australia
(Professor Seeman is the 2002 winner of the prestigious Fredrick C. Bartter Award
of the American Society for Bone and Mineral Research)

*Today's patients want to understand their disease and share actively in
management decisions. (Other) sources of information often leave many
questions unanswered.* The Intelligent Patient Guide to Osteoporosis
*provides a fully-comprehensive, clear and practical account of osteoporosis
and its management that leaves no stone unturned and enables the patient
to understand not only their disease but also its scientific basis. Drs. Sutton
and Josse have produced a unique resource that will both ... educate ...
and empower (patients) to better manage their disease.*

— Professor Juliet Compston, MD FRCP
Professor of Bone Medicine
Cambridge University School of Medicine
Cambridge, UK

... bridges the divide between the physician and the patient. ... (Osteoporosis) is increasingly recognized as a major cause of disability with advancing age. Despite this, many patients go untreated. I hope this book will increase awareness of this eminently treatable disorder and provide useful information for affected patients.

— John Kanis
Emeritus Professor
Director, WHO Collaborating Centre for Metabolic Bone Diseases
University of Sheffield Medical School
President, International Osteoporosis Foundation

An excellent overview of bone health and osteoporosis. This book empowers the reader by providing accurate, unbiased clinical information, including a comprehensive guide through the minefield of pharmacotherapy options for disease management. A welcome addition to our library.

— Sue North, RN MSN
Nurse Clinician
Osteoporosis Program
BC Women's Health Centre
Vancouver, BC

I think this book is really quite outstanding. It is very comprehensive, up-to-date and beautifully-written ... you covered everything I could imagine ... Medical students would do very well with this, and frankly if primary care docs read this, they would be very well served ... this book will both enlighten and empower.

— Ethel S. Siris, MD
Madeline C. Stabile Professor of Clinical Medicine
Columbia University
Director, Toni Stabile Osteoporosis Center
Columbia University Medical Center and New York – Presbyterian Hospital
New York, NY 10032

Although ... written for patients, I would suggest that it is essential reading for (all) health care professionals who treat patients with osteoporosis...

— Barry O. Kassen, MD FRCPC
General Internist
St. Paul's Hospital
Vancouver, BC

This ... comprehensive book will educate and empower patients and families of patients with osteoporosis ... also an excellent review and teaching resource for physicians and other health care professionals who deal with osteoporosis.

— Keith Hatlelid, MD CCFP
Clinical Associate Professor
Department of Family Practice
University of British Columbia

... for the person who wants more than the usual explanations (of) osteoporosis given to patients. ... Diet, exercise, and other preventive measures are clearly presented, and the available drug therapies of osteoporosis are well explained ... an excellent resource for patients and their care-givers.

— David A. Hanley, MD FRCPC
Past Chair, Osteoporosis Canada Scientific Advisory Board
President, Canadian Society of Endocrinology and Metabolism
Professor, Departments of Medicine, Oncology,
and Community Health Sciences
University of Calgary

Having lived with osteoporosis ... since my mid-30s, I lapped up the information in this book. It is unbiased, incredibly comprehensive, (and) easy-to-read and absorb ... information I have struggled to glean from the medical community and personal reading for over 8 years. It is rare to find a book (for patients) written in such an objective manner.

— Sarah McKee
Human Resources Manager and Osteoporosis patient

... my mother was experiencing severe back pain... no one seemed to be able to diagnose or treat her back pain successfully ... we were losing hope ... Dr. Sutton (recognized osteoporosis) and helped her manage her pain and live a more productive life. I found The Intelligent Patient Guide to Osteoporosis *very informative and easy to understand.*

— Ember Schira
Daughter of Patient

We welcome this very informative resource for people whose lives are often dramatically impacted by osteoporosis. The authors are on the forward edge of today's thinking about ... osteoporosis ...

— Dr. Famida Jiwa, MHSc CHE D.C. BSc (Hons)
Vice President, Operations
Osteoporosis Canada

Drs. Sutton and Josse have succeeded admirably. This book ... describes in detail what patients might expect from the modern treatment of osteoporosis.

— Anthony B. Hodsman, MD FRCPC
Professor, Department of Medicine
Division of Nephrology
St. Joseph's Health Care London
London, Ontario

General Praise for *The Intelligent Patient Guide* series of patient-oriented health books

The Intelligent Patient Guide *has been at my side for the last eight months as I fought breast cancer. When I needed (information), it never failed me.*

> — Former CEO Canadian Cancer Society and
> National Cancer Institute of Canada

We learned more from this book than from seven years of dealing with doctors.

> — Patient

The Intelligent Patient Guide to Breast Cancer *walks you through each step of your diagnosis, treatment and prognosis ... with explanations that are easily understood. It brought everything together, making it so clear.*

> — J. McIntosh, Patient

One of the best explanations of breast cancer risk I've seen in print ... dispels the 'panic' of the '1 in 9' statistics. It's lovely to see in print many of the teachings we use on a daily basis.

> — Barbara Warren, RN
> Director of Nursing
> CancerCare Manitoba

As a patient advocate and breast cancer survivor, I lend and use my copy of The Intelligent Patient Guide *often. The book helps equip patients to better understand the need to take charge in the design of their own survival.*

> — B. Cameron

It was so informative. I felt so secure knowing what was going to happen with every step.

> — D. Powell, Patient

A tremendous tool that I make available to all my patients.

> — Dr. J. Caines,
> Halifax, Nova Scotia

I found The Intelligent Patient Guide *an excellent tool during my recent surgery and treatments. It gave me a sense of being an active participant on the road to recovery.*

— S. Moorhouse, RN, Patient

Thank you for writing The Intelligent Patient Guide to Breast Cancer. *It is straightforward and easy to understand. Specific passages particular to my own situation were easily found. It is a most convenient clarification for myself, family and friends.*

— D. Clarke, Patient

This book's clear, concise descriptions and especially its empathetic style made it my only "book" companion along the road of my treatments. I became not only informed but also reassured and calmed.

— H. Thompson, Patient

The Intelligent Patient Guide *is the answer to prayers for making sense of what is happening.*

— D. Sizemore, Patient Spouse

It was my oncologist who first suggested this priceless book ... and it has been a great help to me.

— Patient

Other books in the *Intelligent Patient Guide*
series include:

The Intelligent Patient Guide to Breast Cancer, 4th edition
by Ivo Olivotto, Karen Gelmon, Urve Kuusk
ISBN 0-9696125-8-3

The Intelligent Patient Guide to Colorectal Cancer, 2nd edition
by Michael E. Pezim, MD, David Owen, MB
ISBN 0-9696125-7-5

The Intelligent Patient Guide to Prostate Cancer, 3rd edition
by S. Larry Goldenberg, MD, Ian M. Thompson, MD
ISBN 0-9696125-5-9

Authors

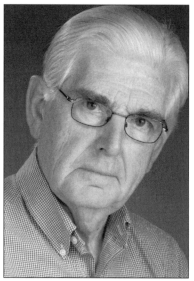

Roger A.L. Sutton, DM FRCPC
Dr. Sutton is a Professor Emeritus of Medicine and Urological Sciences at the University of British Columbia (UBC). He is a past Head of the Division of Nephrology at UBC, past Head of the Department of Medicine at the Vancouver General Hospital and Past President of the Canadian Society of Nephrology. He was Dean of Health Sciences at the Aga Khan University in Karachi, Pakistan, from 1996-2000. Dr. Sutton received his medical training at Oxford University, and his postgraduate training in London and at McGill University in Montreal. He is a Fellow of the Royal Colleges of Physicians of Canada and London, and a Fellow of the American College of Physicians. His research has mainly been in basic and clinical aspects of calcium metabolism.

Editor: Cheryl Edwards MA
Series Editor: Michael E Pezim MD FRCSC
Project Coordinator: Nicola Sutton MBA LLB
Illustrator: Vicky Earle
Manuscript Preparation: Fiona Burrows and Amanda Lee deLeeuw
Design: Peter Woods @ POP Creative
Graphic Production: Angela G. Atkins

Authors

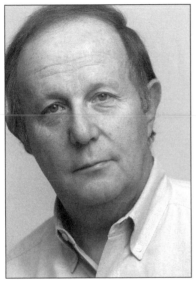

Robert G. Josse, MB BS FRCPC
Dr. Josse is a Professor of Medicine and Nutritional Sciences at the University of Toronto. He is both the past Head of the Division of Endocrinology and Metabolism and Associate Physician-in-Chief at St. Michael's Hospital University of Toronto, and past President of the Canadian Society of Endocrinology and Metabolism. He is the former Chair of the Scientific Advisory Council of Osteoporosis Canada (formerly the Osteoporosis Society of Canada) and is Director of the Osteoporosis Centre at St Michael's Hospital in Toronto. Dr. Josse received his medical training at the University of London (UK), and his postgraduate training in London and at the University of Toronto and the Massachusetts General Hospital in Boston. He is a Fellow of the Royal Colleges of Physicians of Canada and London, and a Fellow of the American College of Physicians. His major research interests include calcium metabolism and osteoporosis.

We dedicate this book to the thousands of patients
living with osteoporosis who, through their courage and curiosity,
have given us the inspiration to write it.

Why read this book?

AS PHYSICIANS WHO HAVE TREATED THOUSANDS OF PATIENTS, we welcome the accessibility of reliable, accurate information on the internet as well as in print. It is refreshing, and sometimes challenging, to encounter a patient in the clinic setting who is knowledgeable about their options, and can ask appropriate questions.

We have put together this osteoporosis guide to act as a personal resource for those interested in this fascinating disease that affects so many of us. If you, or someone close to you, has osteoporosis or is concerned about developing it, this book is for you.

Osteoporosis is a progressive, symptomless deterioration of the bone, which leads to an increased risk of fractures, most often in the wrist, spine and hip. Osteoporosis in older women has received a great deal of emphasis, but it is also common in men, and can occur earlier in life.

Fortunately, there have been major advances in our understanding of bones, how they normally remain strong and healthy, and what we can do about it if osteoporosis develops. All of this is reviewed in detail so that you will be better able to understand the causes, diagnosis and treatment of osteoporosis. Where controversies persist, and they do, they will be carefully described. You will come to know the full range of what is currently understood and what areas need additional research.

As with any disorder, patients do better, both psychologically and often physically, when they understand what is happening. A large part of that is knowing enough to be able to ask questions and take part in the decisions that must be made in osteoporosis prevention and treatment.

- Can diet (calcium and vitamin D) and exercise prevent or reverse osteoporosis?
- If my mother or father has osteoporosis does that increase my risk?
- Should I have my bone mineral density (BMD) measured?
- How great is my risk of fracturing a bone, especially my hip?
- If I need drug treatment, how do I choose which one?
- How do I know if the treatment is working, and what follow-up do I need?

The Intelligent Patient Guide to Osteoporosis answers all of these questions, based on the latest scientific information, and on the experience of our many years of treating patients with osteoporosis in university hospital and community settings.

This guide is about empowering you to take charge of your health. By picking it up and examining it, you have already taken your first step forward. Congratulations. If you choose to read on you will be that much further ahead. We wish you luck on your journey to good health.

Roger Sutton and Robert Josse

Table of contents

PART ONE | **Osteoporosis: What is it and how is it detected?**

The normal skeleton and bone

CHAPTER ONE

The composition of bone

IN ADDITION TO ITS FAMILIAR MECHANICAL FUNCTIONS, the skeleton has a role in providing for the storage of calcium. The bones are a necessary part of the normal motor function of the limbs, where they act as levers in conjunction with muscles. The bones of the pelvis, spine and chest provide support, as well as protection, for internal organs. Likewise, the skull provides essential protection for the brain.

Collagen

The human skeleton is admirably suited to serve both calcium storage and mechanical functions. Bone comprises mineral crystals consisting of apatite, a complex form of calcium phosphate containing small amounts of other substances including hydroxide and carbonate, together with protein, mostly collagen. Bone collagen consists of a tough network of collagen fibers which consist of bundles of collagen molecules (see Figure 1). Each collagen molecule has the form of a triple helix (a twist of three collagen chains). There are cross-links within and between the collagen molecules of bone (which differ from those of collagen in the soft tissues of the body, such as skin).

As collagen is assembled during bone formation, small fragments at the ends of the individual collagen chains, known as

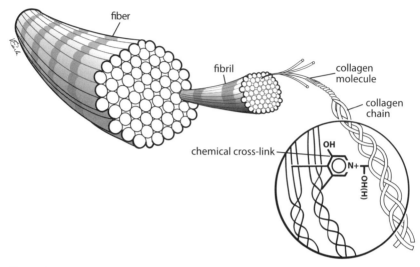

Figure 1: Diagrammatic structure of a collagen fiber
The collagen fiber consists of fibrils, in turn composed of individual collagen collagen molecules (triple helices) which are interconnected through chemical cross links. When collagen is broken down by osteoclasts during bone resorption, these cross links are released into the blood and excreted into the urine, where they can be measured to provide an index of bone resorption.

propeptides, are released into the blood and excreted in the urine. During bone resorption or breakdown, cross-links and their adjacent protein fragments (called telopeptides) are similarly released into the blood and excreted in the urine. The measurement of these collagen fragments, known as "biochemical markers" of bone formation and bone resorption, in blood and/or urine has been useful in studying osteoporosis and its treatment.

The apatite (bone mineral) crystals are arranged on the collagen fiber, the combination giving the bone its normal hard, but not too brittle, consistency.

A great deal of what we know about bone (and indeed about medicine in general) has been revealed by accidents of nature, which we refer to as mutations. An interesting example of this phenomenon is the condition of extreme osteoporosis in early childhood, known as osteogenesis imperfecta. Children with this condition may be born with multiple fractures sustained in the uterus or during delivery. In most individuals with osteogenesis imperfecta, the cause is a mutation in the gene for one of the collagen chains. This particular mutation illustrates the importance of normal collagen as a component of normal strong bones.

Cortical and trabecular bone

The bone of the skeleton is of two major types, so-called cortical and trabecular (cancellous or spongy) bone.

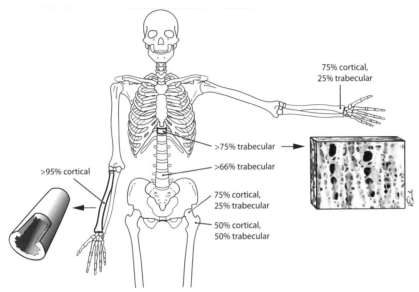

75% cortical, 25% trabecular

>75% trabecular

>66% trabecular

>95% cortical

75% cortical, 25% trabecular

50% cortical, 50% trabecular

Figure 2: The skeleton, showing cortical and trabecular bone
The long bones, such as the humerus in the upper arm, the radius and ulna in the forearm and the femur in the thigh consist mainly of a cylinder of dense cortical bone. Trabecular (spongy) bone is the main component of the vertebral bodies of the spine and is surrounded by a thin shell of cortical bone. The hip region comprises both cortical and trabecular bone.

The cortical bone provides strength and rigidity to the shafts of the long bones.

In trabecular bone, the trabeculae (struts) are arranged to provide maximum strength in the direction of anticipated strains. For example, the greatest strain on the vertebrae results from vertical compression forces. The trabeculae are mainly arranged vertically, with horizontal inter-connections ("ties") which help to prevent buckling.

CHAPTER TWO

Bone remodeling

BONES ARE OFTEN THOUGHT OF AS DRY, or static and unchanging, but like all other tissues of the body, they undergo continuous replacement throughout life.

The process of removal of old bone, and its replacement with new bone, serves several functions. During growth, it allows for modeling (or re-shaping) of the bones, so that, over time, they can enlarge and change in shape to fit the growing child or adolescent.

After we stop growing, the process of remodeling serves to replace areas of microscopic damage such as stress micro-fractures, and probably also helps to maintain conditions in the bone that permit it to function as an immediate source of calcium when needed. The understanding of bone remodeling came originally from the microscopic examination of bone biopsies, which involve the removal of a small fragment or core of bone, under a local anesthetic.

Bone remodeling (or bone multicellular) units

Remodeling occurs in discrete tiny regions of bone, both cortical and trabecular, throughout the skeleton. These microscopic areas of remodeling are known as bone remodeling units (BRUs), or bone multicellular units. In trabecular bone, the BRUs begin as excavations on the surface of trabeculae, whereas inside dense cortical bone, they occur as a cylindrical excavation, sometimes called a "cutting cone". BRUs involve certain cells whose function is to remove the old bone (osteoclasts) and others (osteoblasts) which lay down new bone to replace that which has been removed.

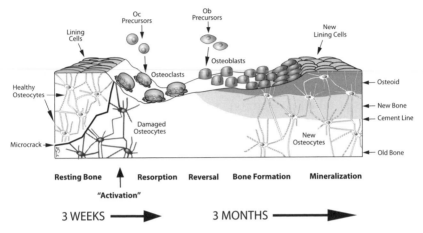

Figure 3: The (trabecular) bone remodeling unit
Bone remodeling in a trabecular bone remodeling unit. Remodeling is necessary to renew bone and repair damage and microcracks. Based on Canalis E et al., Mechanisms of Anabolic Therapies for Osteoporosis. New England Journal of Medicine, 2007, 357, 905-16.

The process of remodeling appears fairly random, but is believed to be targeted in part to areas of micro-damage. Normally, the new bone being added is precisely equal in quantity to that which has been removed, and so the total bone mass remains constant. There is some form of coupling between the osteoclasts (that do the removing) and the osteoblasts (that do the rebuilding), which is critically important but is still not fully understood. A defect in coupling, whereby the bone deposited by the osteoblasts is less than was removed by osteoclasts, is believed to be important in the development of osteoporosis. Most drug treatments for osteoporosis are aimed at altering coupling in the direction of reducing osteoclastic removal of bone (antiresorptive drugs) and/or increasing the osteoblastic addition of new bone (anabolic drugs) in individual remodeling units.

The life cycle of a BRU involves a number of steps, including the formation and activation of osteoclasts, localized bone removal, and the eventual demise of the osteoclast through programmed cell death (known as apoptosis). This is followed by the formation and activation of osteoblasts, which are responsible for the new bone formation. Bone formation begins with the production of collagen, upon which apatite crystals are then deposited, and concludes with the "retirement" of the osteoblasts.

There are three potential fates for osteoblasts: they can die (apoptosis), they can transform into inactive lining cells, or they can become entombed within newly formed bone as cells known as osteocytes. This whole sequence in an individual bone remodeling unit may take between four and eight months. Thereafter there is a quiescent period averaging perhaps two to three years before another remodeling unit occurs in the same area.

An average of about 15% of the bone is undergoing remodeling at any given time, but this is very variable. There are conditions in which remodeling is accelerated, and others in which bone remodeling units are abnormally few in number throughout the skeleton. Accelerated remodeling rates may be an important contributing cause of some types of osteoporosis, such as postmenopausal osteoporosis. Osteoclastic removal of bone from critical locations, such as thin trabeculae, can create weak points where microfractures and trabecular perforations may occur.

Control of osteoclasts and osteoblasts

There is intense interest in understanding how osteoclasts and osteoblasts are regulated, in part because improved understanding of these processes is likely to lead to new and better ways to treat osteoporosis, and perhaps other bone diseases.

Osteoclasts

Osteoclasts are unique cells with several nuclei. Almost all other cells in the human body have a single nucleus. Bone removal is always caused by osteoclasts, which must therefore be playing a key role in the development of osteoporosis.

Osteoclast formation and activation

Osteoclasts are derived from precursor cells in the bone marrow known as macrophages, several of which fuse to form an osteoclast. Osteoclast activity is affected by the level of circulating hormones (including parathyroid hormone, calcitonin and Vitamin D) that will be described later.. Most of the currently available drug treatments for osteoporosis—the so-called antiresorptive drugs—work by decreasing the activity of osteoclasts so that bone turnover (remodeling) decreases. The control of osteoclast formation and activation at the cellular level is complex, and involves a number of locally acting proteins. It is described in Appendix I for readers who may wish to have a little more detail.

Osteoclast function

The process of local bone removal by osteoclasts involves the creation of a seal between the osteoclast and the bone surface, so that the intervening space can be altered chemically in a way that dissolves the bone. This is known to involve the secretion of enzymes into the sealed space, which break down the collagen. In addition, the space can be made very acidic, which dissolves the apatite (calcium phosphate) crystals. There are several inherited disorders in which the bones are abnormally dense. One of these disorders is caused by a mutation of the gene for a protein that is required for the acidification of the space under the osteoclasts, and hence the osteoclasts are unable to remove bone normally. Another inherited disorder in which the bones are too dense, and which is associated with dwarfism, is caused by mutations of the gene for the major enzyme that breaks down collagen (cathepsin K). The artist Toulouse Lautrec is believed to have suffered from this condition.

Osteoblasts

Osteoblasts are the cells that are responsible for laying down new bone, including both the collagen fiber network and the apatite crystals. They are derived from parent cells within the bone marrow.

Osteoblast formation and activation

After local bone removal by osteoclasts has been completed, the osteoclasts undergo programmed cell death (apoptosis) and disappear from the scene. A coupling signal, the nature of which is still not entirely clear, summons osteoblast precursors (which are derived from bone marrow stem cells) to the location where bone has been removed. Osteoporosis treatments that work by increasing osteoblast activity are known as anabolic treatments, in contrast to the antiresorptive treatments that work by reducing osteoclast activity. The control of osteoblast formation and activation, like that of osteoclasts, is complicated and is described in Appendix II for readers who may want a little more information.

Osteoblast function

Active osteoblasts line the surface of the bone in the area resorbed by osteoclasts. Elsewhere the bone is lined with inactive lining cells. The active osteoblasts contain large amounts of the enzyme alkaline phosphatase – one of the markers of bone formation that can be monitored in the blood. Active osteoblasts go through several stages of maturation, during which they secrete bone matrix proteins, particularly collagen, followed by proteins which promote the orderly mineralization of the collagen through deposition of apatite crystals. The crystals are initially rather irregular, but grow and become more uniform as they mature.

The first phase of production of new mineralized bone in a BRU is called primary mineralization, and is completed within weeks. It is followed by a further slow consolidation of bone, during which bone mineral density increases further—so-called secondary mineralization. It is secondary mineralization that, in part, accounts for the increase in bone mineral density when osteoporosis is treated with pure antiresorptive drugs (bisphosphonates that will be discussed later). There is no increase in new bone formation, but a decrease in remodeling, and therefore a reduction in the space occupied by BRUs (the remodeling space), together with progression of secondary mineralization.

As mentioned above, there are several possible fates for osteoblasts. Some become the inactive bone lining cells, some undergo programmed cell death, and some are surrounded by the newly forming bone and transformed into osteocytes, becoming buried within mineralized bone. Osteocytes are in direct communication with each other and with surface osteoblasts and lining cells to form a network, whose main function is believed to be to sense mechanical forces within bone, and respond to them. They may be involved with modeling and remodeling in bone, perhaps helping to direct bone remodeling units towards areas of microdamage.

CHAPTER THREE

Bone changes during life

DURING CHILDHOOD THE SKELETON IS GROWING and the bones are changing shape (modeling) as well as remodeling. At around 20 years of age (in the early third decade), the bone mineral density reaches its maximum—the peak bone mass—earlier in girls than boys, and thereafter, bone mineral density declines with age, particularly after the age of 40.

The major determinant of peak bone mass is probably the family history (genetics), but it can also be influenced by diseases in early life, such as intestinal diseases that affect calcium and/or vitamin D absorption (for example celiac disease), and by medications such as glucocorticoids (given, for example, to treat asthma or childhood arthritis or inflammatory bowel disease). An insufficient dietary intake of calcium and/or vitamin D during childhood would also be expected to limit the achievement of peak bone mass, as would delayed puberty. The absence of menstrual periods, associated with inadequacy of the sex hormones estrogen and progesterone, can seriously impair the development of a normal peak bone mass.

After the peak bone mass has been reached, bone mineral density declines only slowly until menopause in women. As estrogen levels decline around the time of menopause, there is a phase of accelerated bone loss, averaging 2–3% per year at the spine, which can be prevented by the administration of estrogen (hormone replacement therapy). This phase of rapid bone loss lasts about five years, and is then followed by a slower decline in bone mineral density averaging 0.5% per year for the remainder of life. Men do not have the rapid postmenopausal loss of bone, but have a more gradual loss which accelerates after the age of about 70 years.

The reason for the accelerated bone loss in women after menopause is the 90% decline in estrogen production by the ovaries. This leads to an increase in bone turnover, with increased frequency of activation of bone remodeling units (BRUs). There is also uncoupling of bone formation and bone removal so that insufficient new bone is formed to replace the old bone that has been removed. The increased turnover magnifies the effect of the uncoupling. Not only does bone mineral density decline, but the activity of the bone remodeling units further increases fracture risk by creating holes (porosity) in cortical bone, and by osteoclastic excavations of trabeculae, which lead to weakening and increased risk of fatigue microfractures, or which may even directly perforate the trabeculae leading to loss of structural integrity.

A   B

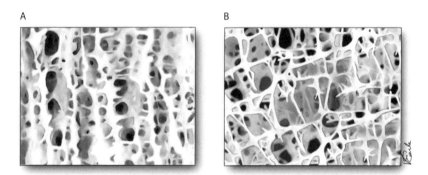

Figure 4 Normal and osteoporotic trabecular bone

Normal (A) and osteoporotic (B) trabecular bone. In contrast to those of the normal bone, the trabeculae in the osteoporotic bone are thinner and frequently lack connectivity where they have been eroded by excessive osteoclastic bone resorption. These changes result in serious weakening of the bone as well as a reduction in bone mineral density.

What is osteoporosis?

CHAPTER FOUR

Osteoporosis

Fragile bones

ANYONE SUFFICIENTLY CURIOUS TO ACCESS A PATIENT GUIDE to osteoporosis probably already knows a little about this disorder, either because of concern for their own health, or for that of a friend or relative. Thanks to considerable research over the past two or three decades, osteoporosis is becoming better understood, and its diagnosis and treatment are improving. As we shall see, however, it is difficult to give a simple and completely satisfactory definition for osteoporosis, but it is instructive to look back at the earliest observations, dating from more than 50 years ago.

Osteoporosis was given its name by German pathologists. The name literally means "porous bones". Because microscopic examination of the bone showed no striking abnormalities, an early description of osteoporosis was "a condition in which there is too little bone, but what there is, is normal". Osteoporosis was recognized to be particularly prevalent in postmenopausal women, in whom it was presumed to result from the precipitous decline in the production of female hormones (progesterone and especially estrogen) that accompanies menopause. This gave rise to the familiar term "postmenopausal osteoporosis", which has tended to obscure the fact that osteoporosis also occurs quite commonly in men, and at earlier ages in both sexes.

In those early days, there were no good diagnostic tests for osteoporosis. The routine tests used to diagnose bone and calcium disorders, such as measurement of the calcium level in the blood and in the urine, gave normal results. Had the disorder simply been a lack of calcium, one might have expected the amount of calcium in the blood or urine to be reduced. Furthermore, it was predicted that calcium, given by a slow intravenous infusion, would be vigorously retained by the body, yet such tests showed that the intravenous calcium was rapidly lost into the urine, at the same rate as in normal, non-osteoporosis subjects, strongly suggesting that osteoporosis was not simply a result of calcium deficiency.

A current accepted definition of osteoporosis is "a generalized condition of the skeleton characterized by compromised bone strength, in which there is a reduced content or "mass" of bone, often associated with deterioration of its fine (microscopic) structure, leading to abnormal fragility and an increased risk of fracturing (breaking) bones".

A common feature of patients with osteoporosis is that they have a reduced bone mineral density (calcium content). This will be described more fully in Chapter 7.

In osteoporosis, so-called fragility fractures may occur with minimal trauma, sometimes so minimal that it is surprising to the patient that a bone could have broken. Fractures in osteoporosis most commonly occur in the hip, the spine (vertebral bodies) and the wrist, but other bones may also suffer fragility fractures, for example the humerus (upper arm) and ribs.

Osteoporosis is painless, unless there is a fracture

An extremely important feature of osteoporosis, and a frequent cause of confusion to patients and their families, is that it is painless. Indeed, it is completely without symptoms, unless or until a fracture occurs. Even then, some osteoporosis fractures are painless. Osteoporosis has sometimes been called "the silent thief", to highlight the fact that it can be developing and progressing quietly, without any awareness on the part of the patient or his or her physician. It should be recognized, however, that some loss of bone is part of the normal aging process.

While it may be a fragility fracture that first draws attention to the presence of osteoporosis, it has been appreciated for many years that an earlier diagnosis would allow effective treatment to be introduced, in order to strengthen the bones and help to prevent fractures. In this respect osteoporosis is similar to some other serious medical conditions, for example high blood pressure. An individual may have high blood pressure which is causing long-term damage to the heart and arteries, in the complete absence of symptoms.

CHAPTER FIVE

How common is osteoporosis and what is its cost to society?

OSTEOPOROSIS IS A VERY COMMON DISORDER, contributing to many fractures, particularly those which occur in older people. Because the population is rapidly aging, this problem is likely to get worse.

Fractures of the hip most commonly result from a fall from a standing height leading to a direct impact on the hip. Both the fall and a reduction in the strength of the bone contribute to the hip fracture. Hip fractures are painful, and lead to admission to hospital, especially of elderly persons, where they are exposed to other serious potential problems such as infections. Approximately one half of patients who were able to walk independently prior to the fracture are unable to do so after the event, even after it has been repaired, so the consequences are significant. In addition, hip fractures are an important contributing cause of death in the elderly. They are also expensive to treat.

Compression fractures of the vertebral bodies of the spine can be painful, but are often painless. Recurrent vertebral compression fractures, affecting several vertebrae, can result in loss of height and forward curvature of the spine (kyphosis), and may ultimately lead to disfigurement and accompanying loss of self-esteem. We still often see older women, and men, who have suffered repeated vertebral compression fractures and have obvious spinal deformities that give them a forward "hunch" in their posture.

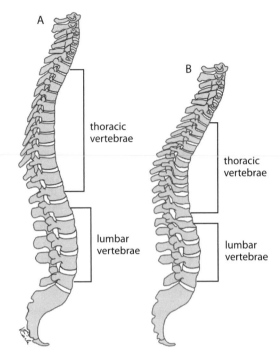

Figure 5: Side, or lateral, view of the spine of (A) a normal individual and (B) a patient with advanced osteoporosis
In the osteoporotic spine many of the individual thoracic and lumbar vertebral bodies have lost their normal rectangular shape and become compressed, leading to substantial loss of height and increased curvature of the spine.

As will be discussed later, available treatments for osteoporosis tend to be more effective in increasing the strength of the vertebrae than the hip, and some recent trials of new treatments have shown very dramatic reductions in the risk of vertebral fracture, giving reason to hope that serious spinal deformities resulting from vertebral compression fractures might soon become a rarity.

Numerous estimates have been published of the number of patients with osteoporosis, the number of fractures attributable to osteoporosis, and the cost of the diagnosis and management of osteoporosis to society. Because there is no universally accepted definition of osteoporosis, these estimates are only very rough approximations, but the numbers are impressive. A recent review suggested that osteoporosis affects 4–6 million women and 1–2 million men in the US. Hip fractures were estimated to cost over $20 billion in the US in 1997. According to Osteoporosis Canada (formerly the Osteoporosis Society of Canada), one in four Canadian women and at least one in eight Canadian men over age 50 have osteoporosis.

The cost of treating osteoporosis and fractures is estimated to be $1.9 billion per year in Canada. Based on hospital discharge data from 1993–1994, the number of hip fractures was estimated at over 23,000, with 1,570 deaths in the acute care setting. These numbers were projected to increase to 88,000 and 7,000 respectively by 2041, highlighting the serious implications unless fracture rates are reduced by some form of intervention. There is some very early evidence suggesting that fracture rates might be beginning to decrease in Canada, perhaps as a result of improved diagnosis and treatment of osteoporosis.

Such recognition of the cost of osteoporosis to society has led to a substantial increase in spending on osteoporosis research in high-income countries over the past two to three decades, which is beginning to bear fruit in the form of improvements in methods for diagnosing osteoporosis, and new treatments. A number of innovative treatments have been introduced recently, and several more are at various phases in the testing process.

CHAPTER SIX

Primary versus secondary osteoporosis

MOST OLDER WOMEN WITH OSTEOPOROSIS have no identifiable explanation for the disorder, although it is believed that heredity plays an important role. These patients are described as having "primary" osteoporosis. Included in this category is the familiar postmenopausal osteoporosis.

Some patients with osteoporosis, particularly men and younger women, have associated medical problems that are known to cause it. These include deficiency of sex hormones (e.g. premature menopause), previous treatment with glucocorticoid medications (e.g. prednisone), over-activity of the parathyroid glands (primary hyperparathyroidism), and excess alcohol consumption.

Recently, the use of certain medications has been shown to be, unexpectedly, associated with an increased risk of fractures. Examples are a new class of drugs for blood sugar control in type 2 diabetes (rosiglitazone and pioglitazone) and proton pump inhibitors which have been very widely used to treat gastroesophageal reflux and peptic ulcer disease. There is great interest in the mechanisms through which an anti-diabetic drug such as rosiglitazone might adversely affect bone. There is increasing evidence that the parent cell (stem cell) in the bone marrow which gives rise to osteoblasts is also the parent of bone marrow fat cells. It appears that rosiglitazone may direct stem cells towards the formation of fat cells rather than osteoblasts.

When osteoporosis is caused by a known disorder it is called "secondary osteoporosis", because it is secondary to something else. Secondary osteoporosis needs to be considered and excluded, sometimes by specific diagnostic tests, before a diagnosis of primary osteoporosis can be made and treatment for primary osteoporosis begun.

The initial assessment of an osteoporosis patient will include a complete medical history and physical examination, measurement of standing height as a baseline, and appropriate laboratory tests to exclude secondary causes of osteoporosis. Specialized clinics may also measure bone turnover markers, urine calcium, vitamin D and parathyroid hormone levels, thyroid and other hormones (testosterone, estradiol, etc.), and rarely (if indicated) a bone biopsy may be done.

Disorders that "sound like" osteoporosis but are not

There are some other medical conditions whose names are similar to osteoporosis and may be confusing to patients. Osteoporosis is sometimes confused with osteoarthritis, but the two conditions are unrelated. *Osteoarthritis* is a painful degenerative disease of joints, often the hips, knees, hands or spine, whereas osteoporosis is a disease of bone which is painless, unless fractures occur.

Osteomalacia is the bone disease that results from severe vitamin D deficiency in adults, as well as from some other rare disorders not directly related to vitamin D deficiency. The bone shows a characteristic delay in the mineralization of newly formed collagen. Dietary osteomalacia is rare in the western world, in part because of vitamin D supplementation of the diet. It is most often seen in patients with disease of the intestine (such as celiac disease) which interferes with the absorption of vitamin D from food. Fractures may occur, often at sites which are unusual in osteoporosis, such as the pelvis. The bones may also be tender to pressure, unlike in osteoporosis where the bones are not tender.

Rickets is the childhood equivalent of adult osteomalacia. Rickets resulting from lack of exposure to sunshine and lack of vitamin D in the diet first appeared when people began to live in cities, and was common in the late 17th century when it became known as the English disease. By the late 18th century fish oil had become a popular cure, but vitamin D itself was not isolated until early in the 20th century. Children with severe rickets have stunting of growth and bony deformities. Nutritional osteomalacia and rickets, as would be expected, can be prevented or cured with adequate vitamin D treatment.

Other causes of a low bone mineral density

Among patients with a reduced bone mineral density, a very small number have a disorder other than primary or secondary osteoporosis, such as generalized malignant (cancerous) bone disease, most commonly multiple myeloma, a leukemia-like disorder of certain cells in the bone marrow. In any patient with suggestive signs or symptoms, appropriate tests should be done to confirm or exclude these serious conditions.

Methods for detecting osteoporosis and determining its severity

CHAPTER SEVEN

The concept of bone mineral density (BMD)

IT IS THE CALCIUM IN BONE which interferes with the transmission of an X-ray beam through the bone, leading to the familiar negative X-ray image of white bones on a black background. Although a plain X-ray may provide suggestive evidence of osteoporosis, it is not accurate enough to be relied upon.

The ability to precisely measure bone quantity or bone mineral density has only become available in the past few decades, through the development and refinement of various types of bone densitometer. Previously, osteoporosis could only be diagnosed after the patient had suffered one or more fractures, or when it was sufficiently advanced to be appreciated on a plain X-ray. This chapter deals mainly with the form of X-ray densitometry which has become the standard way of diagnosing and assessing the degree of osteoporosis—the dual photon X-ray absorptiometry test, or DXA.

Plain X-rays

Most patients who have had a fracture will have had X-rays of the damaged bones. X-rays performed for this or other reasons, such as those of the chest, spine and abdomen, also show parts of the skeleton. In severe osteoporosis, the radiologist examining the X-ray may comment that the bones appear "osteoporotic" (less dense than normal). However, routine X-rays are not intended to assess bone mineral density, and the radiologist's subjective impression is not always correct. The radiologist may also note the incidental presence of a vertebral (spinal) compression fracture, which may be old or recent, and may or may not have caused any symptoms.

In the pre-bone densitometry era, plain X-rays of the spine repeated over time, particularly a side (lateral) view, were the principal way of assessing progress in the patient with osteoporosis. The presence of a vertebral fracture has important implications, being associated with a substantially increased risk of further vertebral fractures and hip fractures. A vertebral compression fracture may range in appearance from a depression of the upper or lower surface of the vertebra, with preservation of the vertical height, to complete crush fractures and major loss of vertebral height. The earliest stages may be difficult to recognize, and are easily overlooked. The process may be gradual, rather than sudden as in other bone fractures, which may help to explain why they may be painless. The discovery of a new vertebral compression fracture has the same significance as any other fragility fracture, and the detection of new vertebral fractures obviously indicates that the treatment is not achieving the desired result.

Since the 1980s, X-ray absorptiometry, has replaced the review of sequential spinal X-rays for the diagnosis and monitoring of osteoporosis. This technique relies upon quantifying the degree of the absorption of X-rays by the calcium in bone to obtain a measurement of the amount of calcium in particular bones. This measurement is known as bone mineral density (BMD).

Bone densitometry

The earliest X-ray bone densitometers were designed for application to the peripheral skeleton, usually the forearm. These single photon absorptiometers (SPAs) had much more limited use than modern dual photon X-ray absorptiometers (DXAs); nevertheless, they showed the potential value of bone mineral density measurements, and were used in many of the early studies.

Single photon absorptiometers were succeeded by dual photon X-ray absorptiometers (DXAs) designed to determine bone mineral density in central sites such as the lumbar vertebrae and the hip, which have greater relevance to clinical osteoporosis. If required, forearm measurements can also be made, but they are not routine. The patient lies on a table and is scanned by the machine. The process takes a few minutes and involves a very small radiation dose. Usually DXA gives a precise and accurate measurement of bone mineral density, but under certain circumstances, bone mineral density may be over- or under- estimated. For example, DXA tends to overestimate bone mineral density in patients with large bones, and underestimate it in those with small bones. Severe arthritis of the spine can result in a spuriously high value for bone mineral density (BMD).

The ability to measure bone mineral density with reasonable precision and reproducibility was an essential requirement both for the accurate diagnosis of osteoporosis, and for the development and monitoring of treatment, and has been central to most of the recent clinical advances in osteoporosis. DXA can also provide an inexpensive radiographic image of the spine, requiring a low radiation dose, which can detect vertebral fractures—so-called vertebral fracture assessment or VFA.

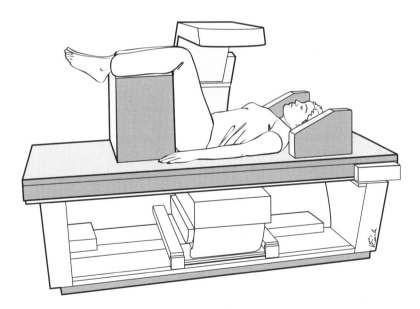

Figure 6: Dual photon X-ray absorptiometer (DXA)
The DXA bone densitometer, designed to measure bone mineral density at the spine and hip. Modern instruments can also provide an X-ray image of the vertebral bodies, viewed from the side, allowing a vertebral fracture assessment (VFA)

The DXA report

The DXA report provides bone mineral density values (expressed as grams per square cm) for various regions of the hip, including the total hip and femoral neck, and for individual lumbar (L) vertebrae, and an average of lumbar vertebrae (usually L 1 to 4 or L 2 to 4. Any vertebra that is fractured or has some other obvious abnormality is excluded. If either the spine or the hip cannot be reported, for example due to multiple vertebral compression fractures or surgical hip replacements, the forearm (radius bone) can be used as an alternative site.

CHAPTER EIGHT

Using T-scores to express severity of osteoporosis

DUAL PHOTON X-RAY ABSORPTIOMETRY measures the amount of mineral in a given area of bone. This gives a bone mineral density in grams per square centimeter. Bone mineral density has been estimated to account for two thirds of the strength of the bones.

By convention, bone mineral densities of the spine and hip are generally reported as "T-scores". This convention arose from a group of specialists at the World Health Organization (WHO), who developed a definition of osteoporosis in 1994 that was intended for use in epidemiological studies—for example studies that make population estimates of the economic consequences of osteoporosis. The definitions were not originally intended for use in managing individual patients.

The group proposed a definition for (postmenopausal) osteoporosis based on the T-score, which is defined as the number of standard deviations by which the measured bone mineral density falls below that of a young (age 20–29) normal Caucasian female (see Appendix III). In older men, the T-score is obtained by comparing the patient with a young adult (Caucasian) man. The standard deviation is a statistical measure of the spread of values within a population.

The World Health Organization group originally recommended that a T-score of minus 2.5 (–2.5) or less at the spine, hip or forearm be used as the cut-off level for diagnosing osteoporosis. In other words, if the patient's T-score at spine, hip or forearm was –2.5 or less, meaning that the bone mineral density was 2.5 or more standard deviations below the average for a young adult, the patient was deemed to have osteoporosis.

The World Health Organization group also described a second diagnostic category, which they called "osteopenia" (meaning less bone than normal), defined as a T-score between –1.0 and –2.5. The term "osteopenia" has led to some confusion amongst patients in that it implies the presence of a disease state when, in fact, there may be none (more about this in Chapter 10).

As might be expected, the determination of bone mineral density at the hip is better for predicting hip fracture than measurements at other sites such as the spine. The risk of hip fracture increases about 2.6 fold for each standard deviation decrease in the hip bone mineral density. That is, a patient with a T-score at the hip of –3.5 has, on average, 2.6 times the risk of sustaining a hip fracture in the next decade compared with a patient with a T-score of –2.5. The risk of any osteoporotic fracture increases about 1.5 fold for each standard deviation decrease in the bone mineral density measurement at other sites.

CHAPTER NINE

Other methods for assessing bone quantity and quality

IN CHAPTER 7, we dealt with dual photon X-ray absorptiometry testing (DXA), which is currently the standard technique for diagnosing and monitoring osteoporosis. In this chapter we describe several other tests that are used to study bone quantity as well as a number of tests that provide information on other aspects of bone such as bone turnover. Many of these tests are not routinely used in clinical practice, but have provided valuable information in research studies of new treatments for osteoporosis.

Ultrasound (QUS)

The use of ultrasound to evaluate bone quality has been under investigation for some years. At first it was hoped that ultrasound might provide a useful measure of bone quality, independent of bone mineral density (DXA) but that has not been proved to be the case. When doing ultrasound testing, the heel (calcaneus) bone is the most commonly used because of its very easy accessibility. Many instruments are being manufactured, and their results are not identical. It is very important to use an instrument which has been properly validated for that specific purpose.

Two parameters can be measured, the speed of transmission of the ultrasound wave through the bone, and the ultrasound attenuation

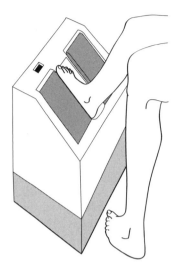

Figure 7:
Quantitative ultrasound (heel) device
Quantitative ultrasound (QUS) device for measuring bone mineral density in the heel bone (calcaneus).

(weakening of the sound waves), which can be combined into a so-called stiffness index, or estimated heel bone mineral density. Attenuation and stiffness are predictive of future hip fracture.

Quantitative ultrasound is substantially less expensive than DXA and in some cities it is being promoted and offered in shopping malls as a simple means of screening for osteoporosis. Although quantitative ultrasound may indeed have significant potential as an inexpensive equivalent of DXA or as a means to improve fracture prediction by DXA, we don't yet know enough about it to accept that it can be relied upon to diagnose osteoporosis accurately. DXA has been the standard for diagnosis and treatment for some years and in most osteoporosis treatment trials, it has been shown that patients who respond to treatment have T-scores by DXA at the hip or spine of less than –2.5. By contrast, a quantitative ultrasound threshold for treatment has not been defined.

It has been suggested that ultrasound might be used for prescreening, in order to determine which patients should have a DXA scan, but earlier evidence suggested that risk factors as determined with a questionnaire might be equally useful in determining who should have DXA. Further studies are being done to determine the optimal role for quantitative ultrasound, both alone and in combination with risk factors, in the diagnosis and management of osteoporosis.

In a recent European study, a group of risk factors was defined which were shown to have predictive value for hip fracture. The predictive value of these risk factors alone was similar to that of quantitative ultrasound (QUS) alone, but the combination was better than either alone. In other words, the combination of risk factors combined with QUS testing had good predictive ability, nearly as good as the new FRAX® assessment (see later).

The main value of QUS testing combined with risk factor assessment may be in jurisdictions, for example rural areas and low income countries, where access to DXA is limited. The combination of QUS testing plus risk factor assessment may allow patients to be triaged into those with obvious osteoporosis needing treatment, those without evidence of osteoporosis (for whom lifestyle measures alone are sufficient), and an intermediate group who could be referred to a larger center for DXA testing.

CT Bone densitometry (QCT)

Computerized tomography (CT scanning) is familiar as a technique used for obtaining images of many internal organs, including the brain and lungs. The CT scan gives an image of a slice through a part of the body. The scanner can be programmed to provide a slice through one or more lumbar vertebrae, and can then select a portion of the slice that includes only the trabecular bone of the vertebral body, excluding the surrounding cortical bone shell. It can then determine an average value for the trabecular bone mineral density of several adjacent vertebrae.

This technique can therefore measure pure trabecular bone mineral density, and follow changes in response to medications. This has proved to be an extremely valuable research tool, but because of cost and the limited access to CT scan machines for non-urgent purposes, it has not become a routine clinical tool. DXA is not able to measure pure trabecular bone—there is always cortical as well as trabecular bone in the path of the X-ray beam that is passing through the spine or hip, and therefore the central bone mineral density determined by DXA represents a combination of cortical and trabecular bone. CT bone densitometry has been very useful in showing that some treatments preferentially affect trabecular bone, which was not apparent from DXA.

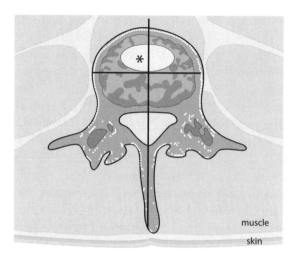

Figure 8: Computerized tomographic (CT) image of a lumbar vertebrae for determination of trabecular bone mineral density
The figure shows a slice through one of the lumbar vertebrae. The instrument is programmed to select a region of pure trabecular bone, avoiding the rim of cortical bone that surrounds it (shown as the ellipse marked with the asterisk), and calculates the average CT density of that selected region.

Nuclear medicine bone scan

The nuclear medicine bone scan employs bone-seeking radioactive material that binds to abnormal areas of bone that then "light up" when the patient is scanned. Nuclear medicine bone scans have traditionally been used mainly for the diagnosis of cancer in the bone and certain other bone diseases. They have a very limited role in osteoporosis. Recent fractures light up on the bone scan, and sometimes this can be useful when it is unclear from the X-ray whether a fracture (usually a compression fracture of a vertebra) is recent or old. An old inactive fracture will not attract the radioactive substance and so will not light up on the scan.

Biochemical markers of bone turnover

As noted earlier, the rate of bone turnover (remodeling) influences bone strength and fracture risk, independently of bone mineral density. Most treatments for osteoporosis alter bone turnover by decreasing bone resorption. Other treatments can increase bone formation or even influence both resorption and formation. As bone turns over as a result of this resorption and formation, proteins and other substances are released into the blood stream. Some of these biochemical markers of bone turnover can be measured in blood or urine samples. They have been very useful in research on osteoporosis, and are occasionally useful in its diagnosis and treatment. The bone mineral density alone does not provide dynamic information on bone turnover, but simply static information on bone mineral density.

Biochemical markers of bone *formation*

The main protein produced by the osteoblast is collagen. However, the osteoblast produces other proteins which are released into the blood, for example the enzyme alkaline phosphatase. Alkaline phosphatase has been measured in the blood for a variety of reasons for many decades and there are other sources of alkaline phosphatase in the blood, including liver, intestine and placenta. Techniques now exist for determining the level of that component of alkaline phosphatase in the blood which has specifically originated from the bone (bone specific alkaline phosphatase), and this is a useful marker of bone formation. Osteocalcin is another protein formed by osteoblasts. It is produced during both bone formation and resorption, and is most useful as an overall indicator of bone turnover.

During osteoblast synthesis of collagen, single chains are assembled into a triple helix and so-called "extension peptides" are clipped off the ends of the individual collagen chains, and released into the blood. Unfortunately these extension peptides are not specific to bone, being formed during the synthesis of skin collagen as well. However, the measurement of these extension peptides (P1CP and P1NP) in the blood can still give some information about bone formation. After the triple helices are assembled, cross-links are formed at intervals between the collagen chains, in part to hold them together (Figure 1). In the management of osteoporosis, bone specific alkaline phosphatase and P1NP, and to a lesser extent osteocalcin, are the most useful markers for bone formation.

Biochemical markers of bone *resorption*

Bone resorption by osteoclasts involves the digestion of collagen by enzymes, resulting in collagen fragments being released into the blood stream and excreted into the urine. The cross links between the collagen chains (Pyd and Dpd), and their associated telopeptides or peptide fragments (NTx and CTx), can be measured in urine, and NTx and CTx can also be measured in blood samples, providing useful indices of bone resorption (Figure 1). Serum CTx is probably the most useful index of resorption in osteoporosis.

• Osteoclasts also produce the enzyme acid phosphatase (TRAP), which can be measured in the blood, and provides another index of bone resorption. All of these markers give somewhat variable results from day to day, and even throughout the day, but they have been very useful in research studies of osteoporosis treatments, and have found some clinical applications. Bone resorption usually drops rapidly with the introduction of an antiresorptive treatment such as a bisphosphonate—the group of drugs that includes alendronate (Fosamax), risedronate (Actonel) and zoledronate, and that are currently the first line treatment for most patients with osteoporosis (discussed in later chapters). Markers of bone resorption can be measured within one month of starting treatment, and if the expected reduction is seen, the patient can be reassured that they are responding to treatment. Failure to respond may indicate that the drug is not being taken correctly; in the case of oral bisphosphonates it may mean that the patient is taking the drug with food or other medications, which are known to interfere with absorption of the drug, and therefore impair its effectiveness.

In some studies, baseline levels of markers have been found to predict responsiveness to the treatment. In the future it is anticipated that levels of markers may help with the choice of treatment in a particular patient.

Bone biopsy

Bone biopsy involves the removal of a small core of bone, usually trabecular bone together with some cortical bone, using a bone biopsy needle and a local anaesthetic. A common site is the iliac crest (pelvic brim) which is readily accessible through the skin.

The small bone sample is put into preservative, then cut into thin sections that are stained and examined under the microscope. It was this technique that led to our present understanding of the role of osteoclasts and osteoblasts in bone remodeling. The bone biopsy is rarely used in routine clinical practice in patients with osteoporosis, in part because it can be painful, and in part because most of the information that is obtained from bone biopsy can now be obtained through non-invasive tests. In osteoporosis, the microscopic appearance of the bone is relatively normal, except that the visible quantity of mineralized bone is less than in the normal non-osteoporotic individual. The trabeculae are thinner than normal, and if the biopsy is very carefully examined, occasional cracks or microfractures may be identified.

The principal indication for a bone biopsy now is uncertainty of the diagnosis. Bone biopsy is helpful in distinguishing osteomalacia from osteoporosis (though a biopsy is not always necessary) and can be useful in diagnosing various malignant diseases of bone. A bone biopsy may be considered if there is any suggestion of one of these conditions from the patient's history, from the physical examination, or from the results of other tests.

An interesting refinement of the bone biopsy is the use of tetracycline markers. Tetracyclines are a family of antibiotics which, for chemical reasons, are deposited in a linear fashion on the surface of bone trabeculae at sites where bone mineralization is occurring at the time the drug is given. Tetracyclines are fluorescent when observed under ultraviolet light. A second tetracycline dose can be given, usually a couple of weeks after the first, followed by the bone biopsy. Microscopic examination of a section of the bone under ultraviolet light then shows the linear tetracycline "labels", and the distance between them indicates the amount of new bone formation that has occurred during the period between the two tetracycline doses. Different tetracyclines which fluoresce with different colors can be given for the first and second label, to facilitate distinguishing between the labels. This ability to measure new bone formation has been very useful in understanding the processes of bone formation and resorption.

Often during the development of new drugs for the treatment of osteoporosis, a sub-set of the patients receiving the drug, as well as a sub-set of subjects receiving placebo, will undergo bone biopsy (having given informed consent), in order to document the effects of the drug on bone at a microscopic level, and ensure that there are no undesirable effects on the bone.

High resolution CT and MRI imaging

As the resolution of CT and MRI scanners improves, it is becoming possible to obtain 3-dimensional images of the fine structure (micro-architecture) of bone, including trabeculae. Until now, only 2-dimensional images derived from bone biopsies were available.

Recent studies with a new "HRpQCT" (high resolution peripheral quantitative CT) scanner that can examine the radius (forearm) bone showed a good correlation between the radius and the iliac crest bone biopsy, including estimated number and thickness of trabeculae. This gives reason to hope that the high resolution CT scan of the radius bone might, in the future, reduce the need for invasive bone biopsy in patients undergoing trials of new osteoporosis treatments.

Studies with HRpQCT at the radius have shown differences in the changes that occur in the trabeculae with aging between men and women. Women tend to undergo loss of trabecular number, while men begin adult life with thicker trabeculae, which become thinner, without loss of trabecular number. These differences in bone quality would not be apparent from measurements of bone mineral density by the standard DXA test. Under certain circumstances, monitoring of treatment by these newer machines may reflect the response to treatment better than DXA.

CHAPTER TEN

Osteopenia versus osteoporosis

A DIAGNOSIS OF OSTEOPOROSIS has traditionally been made when the patient's T-score falls below a threshold of minus 2.5 (−2.5). A T-score in the range of −1.0 to −2.5 has been called "osteopenia", meaning less bone than normal. However, the label osteopenia should not be interpreted as indicating the presence of a disease—many such individuals may have an acceptable bone mineral density.

Problems with "osteopenia" versus "osteoporosis"

The confusion regarding the term osteopenia illustrates an important limitation of T-scores, namely that their significance depends on other factors, particularly the patient's age. The T-score compares the patient's bone mineral density (BMD) with average values of *young normal persons* and therefore it is not surprising that most elderly patients have a negative T-score, many of them below −1.0, the threshold for "osteopenia". Because bone density normally declines with age, a much larger proportion of normal people fall in the osteopenic range at age 70 than at age 40 (see Appendix III). In reality, many such individuals labeled as "osteopenic" actually have an acceptable bone mineral density *for their age*. It is now felt that it would be better not to create the impression that they have a "disease", but rather to describe the bone mineral density in some other way, preferably in terms of the estimated future risk of fracture (see Chapter 11).

In younger people, an alternative method of reporting DXA results has been developed. It is called the Z-score system. In the Z-score system, the patient's bone mineral density is compared with that of age- and sex-matched normal subjects. Z-scores are now used when testing premenopausal women (see Appendix III) and in men under 50 years of age. The reason they are not used in older people lies in the difficulty in defining older people who are known to be free of osteopenia and osteoporosis. Since these conditions are so common amongst older persons, it is difficult, if not impossible, to obtain reliable age- and sex-matched normal bone mineral density values with which the patient's bone mineral density can be compared to obtain a Z-score.

Although the definitions of osteoporosis and osteopenia were derived by comparison with young Caucasian women, there are data supporting the applicability of these same cut-off numbers to men. For example, men suffer increasing numbers of hip fractures at similar bone mineral densities and T-scores as do women. However, there are only limited data on the applicability of these criteria to non-Caucasian ethnic groups.

As already noted, the distinction between osteoporosis and osteopenia is somewhat arbitrary. In a US population study of 150,000 postmenopausal women, 6% were classified as having osteoporosis, while 39% had osteopenia on the basis of their T-scores. Because there are so many more individuals with osteopenia than osteoporosis (about six times as many), the total number of fractures is actually larger among individuals with osteopenia than osteoporosis. Furthermore, bone mineral density measurement alone has a very low sensitivity as a predictor of fracture—less than 5% of women suffering a fracture between 50 and 60 years of age would have been diagnosed as having osteoporosis on the basis of T-scores had they been tested at age 50. This very limited ability to predict fractures is one of the reasons why population screening of women with DXA at the time of menopause is not widely recommended.

Because of the limitations of using T-scores and the arbitrary classification as osteopenia or osteoporosis, there has been an ongoing effort for several years to develop an estimate of the absolute risk of future fracture, to improve the diagnosis and treatment of osteoporosis. The results of this work are described in the next chapter.

CHAPTER ELEVEN

Risk of fracture: The FRAX® risk calculator

THE PRINCIPAL RISK OF OSTEOPOROSIS, which one would wish to avert by treatment, is fractures. We have seen that the T-score alone is not a good predictor of future fracture.

Several factors determine whether a patient will suffer a fracture. Age is a very important determinant of fracture risk, independent of the T-score *(see figure 9 on next page)*. Possible reasons for this age effect include an increased risk of falls in the elderly, as well as changes in bone quality with aging. Other factors which are well recognized to independently increase the risk of fracture are glucocorticoid use and a history of previous fragility fractures.

Many jurisdictions have been trying to develop fracture risk assessments to guide clinical management. For example, Osteoporosis Canada's 10-year fracture risk assessment utilizes bone mineral density, age and sex as well as history of fragility fracture or glucocorticoid use, to score the patient's 10-year fracture probability as low (<10%), moderate (10–20%) or high (>20%). It should be recognized that absolute risk assessments are only applicable to untreated patients.

Fracture Risk Assessment Tool (FRAX®)

The World Health Organization 10-year fracture risk project is a very large study using population data from North America,

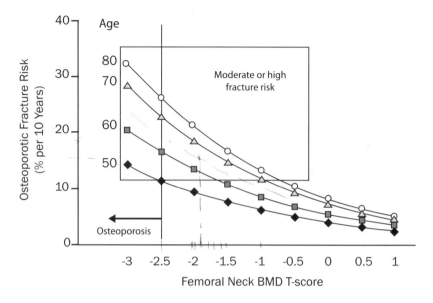

Figure 9: The impact of age on absolute fracture risk at different measured bone mineral densities at the hip (femoral neck)

A T-score of –2.0 confers a 10% risk of fracture within 10 years in a 50-year-old woman, whereas in an 80-year-old woman, a T-score of –0.5 is associated with a similar 10-year fracture risk. Stated differently, a T-score of –2.5 confers a 10-year fracture risk of about 10% at age 50, and over 25% at age 80. This figure illustrates why the use of a T-score of –2.5 to define osteoporosis, without reference to the patient's age or other relevant risk factors, is of limited usefulness. Ten Year Probabilities of Osteoporotic Fractures According to BMD and Diagnostic Thresholds. Kanis JA et al., Osteoporosis International, 2001, 12, 989–995

Europe, Asia and Australia, designed to identify and assign weight to all of the important independent risk factors for fracture, so that they can be integrated into an index of 10-year fracture risk (with or without a bone mineral density measurement). This project has recently generated a Fracture Risk Assessment Tool (FRAX®) *http://www.shef.ac.uk/FRAX*, for the UK and several other European countries, China and the United States.

Risk factors used in computing the FRAX® 10-year fracture risk include, in addition to age and gender:

1. Body mass index or BMI (derived from height and weight and expressed in kilograms per square meter). Specifically,

leanness is a risk factor for hip fracture, partly attributable to bone mineral density.

2. History of fragility fracture, especially recurrent vertebral fracture.
3. Parental history of fragility fracture, especially hip.
4. Current cigarette smoking.
5. Long-term glucocorticoid use.
6. Alcohol use, three or more drinks per day.
7. Rheumatoid arthritis, which confers a risk over and above bone mineral density.
8. Causes of secondary osteoporosis including hypogonadism (inadequate sex hormone levels), chemotherapy for breast cancer, inflammatory bowel disease, prolonged immobility, organ transplantation, type 1 diabetes, thyroid disease (hyperthyroidism).

Each additional positive risk factor incrementally increases fracture probability by a specific amount; some risk factors are stronger than others.

The fracture risk for several jurisdictions in Europe, North America and elsewhere can be computed directly through the FRAX® web site. The application of the FRAX® risk calculator to clinical practice is currently being very actively explored, both to assess fracture probability, and to help in determining who should have bone mineral density testing. This information can then be used to guide treatment decisions.

The FRAX® risk calculator is expected to be incorporated into bone mineral density measurement software, and will be included in clinical reports. It is intended for use in postmenopausal women and men aged 50 and older who have not received treatment for osteoporosis.

The National Osteoporosis Foundation (NOF) of the US currently recommends that postmenopausal women and men age 50 or over presenting with the following should be recommended for treatment:

- A hip or vertebral fracture;
- T-score equal to or less than –2.5 at the femoral neck or spine after appropriate investigation to exclude secondary causes;
- Low bone mass (T-score between –1.0 and –2.5 at the femoral neck or spine and a 10-year probability of a hip fracture

greater than 3% or a 10-year probability of a major osteo-porosis-related fracture greater than 20% based on the US-adapted FRAX® algorithm.

Each jurisdiction will need to develop its own recommenda-tions, which will need to take into account local factors such as the costs of investigation and treatment versus the benefits obtained. Studies are underway in several jurisdictions to determine what proportion of the population of postmenopausal women and men over 50 would be treated using the FRAX® criteria, and whether these proportions are economically and clinically appropriate. For example in the US, guidelines based on estimates of fracture probability using FRAX® would result in the recommendation to treat 73% of Caucasian women over 65 and 90% over 75 years of age.

Some patients with a high fracture risk can be treated without the need for a bone mineral density measurement. Where the risk is not so high, a bone mineral density measurement will be required, and there are data to suggest that the appropriate thresh-old bone mineral density for treatment may be different according to which positive risk factors are present. For example, there are data to support treatment at a bone mineral density of −1.0 or less in a patient with a family history of hip fracture, whereas for the weaker risk factors such as smoking or excess alcohol, the current treatment threshold of −2.5 or less may be appropriate.

As physicians and other health care workers get used to using and interpreting 10-year fracture risk, this index will increasingly be used as an assessment and treatment tool. Local data, including those pertaining to health economics and cost effectiveness, will be needed to adapt the tool to different jurisdictions. In the future, other risk factors may be considered for inclusion into the fracture assessment, such as QUS (ultrasound), or biochemical bone mark-ers, but at present there are insufficient data to show that they have independent predictive value.

Examples of the application of the FRAX® tool

A few examples illustrate the magnitude of the effect of taking risk factors into account, as well as an example obtained with FRAX® in the presence or absence of a bone mineral density measurement.

1. 10-year hip fracture probability is 100-times higher in an 80-year-old with a parental history of hip fracture than in a 50-year-old with no risk factors.
2. In a 65-year-old woman the 10-year hip fracture probability in the absence of risk factors is 2.3% at a BMI (body mass index) of 20 kg/m2 but four times lower (0.6%) at a BMI of 40 kg/m2.
3. A 65-year-old female with a BMI of 25 and no risk factors has a 10-year risk of osteoporotic fracture of 8.6%, and of hip fracture of 1.3%. A history of previous fragility fracture increases these to 16.4 and 3.2% respectively. In each of these examples, a measured bone mineral density at the osteoporosis threshold of –2.5 changes these risks to 12.4 and 3.0% and 20.2 and 5.0% respectively—higher than in the absence of the bone mineral density measurement, but similar overall risks.

Recommendations of Osteoporosis Canada for bone mineral density assessment

It is anticipated that the FRAX® tool may be used in the future to determine who should have a bone mineral density determination. In the meantime, many jurisdictions have developed their own guidelines for determining who should have a bone mineral density test. Table 1 lists the current recommendations of Osteoporosis Canada.

Table 1   **Recommendations of Osteoporosis Canada regarding who should have a bone mineral density measurement**
Age 65 or older
Risk factor assessment indicates high risk
Loss of 4 or more cm in height overall, or 2 or more cm in one year
Presence of kyphosis – a hump or excessive curvature of the back
Taking long-term glucocorticoid medication
Recent fracture in which osteoporosis is suspected (to make decisions regarding further diagnosis and treatment options)
Monitoring effectiveness of treatment for established osteoporosis

The recommendations of other groups such as the International Osteoporosis Federation (IOF) and the International Society for Clinical Densitometry (ISCD) for bone mineral density testing can be obtained from their respective websites (*www.iofbonehealth.org* and *www.iscd.org*).

Understanding bone metabolism

CHAPTER TWELVE

Calcium

THE NORMAL ADULT HUMAN BODY contains approximately one kg of calcium, of which 99% is located in bone, where it is present mainly as crystals of apatite, a form of calcium phosphate.

The remaining 1% of calcium in the body, outside the bone, serves many essential functions. Calcium is required for, and is critical in the regulation of, many body functions including the transmission of nerve impulses, muscle and heart contractions and hormone secretion by endocrine glands.

In health, the calcium concentration in the blood is kept within a very narrow normal range, between 2.10 and 2.55 mmol/litre (8.4 – 10.2 mg/100 ml), despite the large exchanges of calcium that normally occur between bone and blood and between the intestine and blood, as dietary calcium is absorbed.

Approximately one half of the calcium in the blood is in the form of free calcium ions (Ca^{++}); the remainder is bound to protein (albumin). It is the free (ionized) calcium that is regulated by the parathyroid glands. Although the free (ionized) calcium level can be measured in the laboratory, it is more expensive and less precise than the total calcium measurement, which usually suffices for clinical purposes.

Calcium, like hydrogen, oxygen and sodium is a chemical element. Although the term "calcium" is often used when discussing osteoporosis, calcium is a very reactive substance which does not exist in nature in a free form, but only as calcium salts such as calcium phosphate or calcium carbonate. However, when describing the calcium content of the diet, or of calcium supplements, it is the quantity of the calcium itself, or elemental calcium (as though it was in free form) that should be noted.

Calcium in the diet

Calcium is an essential constituent of the human diet. In typical western diets, dairy products are the main source of calcium. Other calcium-fortified foods such as orange juice or soy milk may contain comparable amounts of calcium. A few other foods are also quite rich in calcium, including canned fish (e.g. sardines or salmon with the bones). In western countries most people choose diets that contain between 300 and 1200 mg of calcium per day. In assessing your own dietary intake of calcium, always focus on *elemental* calcium.

Appendix IV provides information on the elemental calcium content of common foodstuffs, and allows you to make a rough estimate of your own daily calcium intake.

How much calcium do we need?

Calcium supplements are the biggest seller in the US dietary supplement industry, with estimated annual sales in 2004 of nearly one billion dollars. Despite many decades of study, the issue of what is an adequate daily calcium intake is still quite controversial. There is no universal agreement on how an adequate intake can best be determined. Nevertheless, there are national recommendations, particularly in developed countries, though they differ from one country to another. The UK recommendation is at least 700 mg of calcium per day for adults, whereas in North America, the recommended dietary calcium intake is 1000–1500 mg per day.

Many (perhaps most) adults fall well below these recommended levels. Four cups of milk per day provide about 1200 mg of calcium, but few adults consume this quantity of dairy products. If your own diet contains substantially less than the recommended dietary calcium, you could either increase your intake of foods containing significant amounts of calcium (usually dairy products) or take calcium supplements in pill or liquid form. There is no evidence that calcium consumed as dairy products or any other food has any significant advantage over calcium taken in the form of supplements.

Calcium supplements: Pros and cons

The least expensive calcium supplement is calcium carbonate (chalk). Calcium carbonate is best taken with food, because in some patients it is not well absorbed when taken on an empty stomach. There is very little evidence that other (usually more expensive) calcium supplements are superior to calcium carbonate, except perhaps in a few unusual circumstances (see later). The different calcium salts used for calcium supplements contain different percentages of elemental calcium, as detailed in Table 2.

Table 2 **Calcium content of different calcium supplements**	
Calcium salt	**Percentage elemental calcium**
Calcium acetate	25.3
Calcium carbonate	40
Calcium citrate	21
Calcium glucoheptonate	8
Calcium gluconate	9
Calcium lactate	13
Calcium phosphate dibasic anhydrous	29
Calcium phosphate dibasic dihydrate	23
Calcium phosphate tribasic	40

Who is at special risk of inadequate calcium intake?

Certain individuals are particularly likely to be consuming very low amounts of calcium, including the elderly (especially if living alone, disabled or institutionalized), and those who avoid dairy products, perhaps because of actual or perceived lactose intolerance. For the latter, calcium supplemented soy products may be an appropriate alternative.

A major issue with calcium supplements is the lack of patient "adherence"—patients frequently stop taking their supplements. Calcium supplements are not particularly pleasant to take, and can cause constipation. This side-effect may be lessened by choosing a calcium supplement that contains magnesium, since magnesium has some laxative effect. There is probably no other good reason for the usual patient with osteoporosis to take extra magnesium. There is no convincing evidence that magnesium supplements per se are of any benefit in osteoporosis.

Adolescents are a particularly problematic group, since they require larger calcium intakes than adults, being at the stage in life when the bones are being rapidly built up to their maximum strength, or peak bone mass. Adolescents' dietary habits may also be erratic, and they tend to prefer soft drinks to milk. This is a group in which judicious calcium supplementation might yield considerable long-term benefits, if adolescents could be persuaded to take them.

Benefits and risks of calcium supplements

Large studies of the value of routine calcium supplements in improving bone mineral density and preventing fractures have produced conflicting results, although the balance of the evidence is positive. Since the evidence for supplementation is modest, it may be best to target those individuals whose diet is low in calcium to ensure their adherence to a calcium supplement, rather than giving supplements routinely to all patients.

Possible cardiovascular risks

Until recently, it was believed that there was little risk to taking calcium supplements in quantities sufficient to achieve the recommended calcium intake. However, a recent study from New Zealand has raised new concerns. This study in healthy postmenopausal women showed significantly more "vascular events"—particularly heart attacks (myocardial infarctions)—in those taking calcium supplements (one gram per day as calcium citrate, taken with meals) compared with those taking a placebo. The finding emerged after the supplements had been given for about two years.

Many of the previous studies of the value of calcium supplements in osteoporosis have not reported vascular events, but some others have shown similar trends to the New Zealand study. It is possible that calcium supplements, by transiently increasing the calcium concentration in the blood, could favor the deposition of calcium in arteries, and hence vascular events. This issue is being intensively studied; somewhat reassuringly, a recent study failed to show an association between calcium supplements and calcification of the coronary arteries.

Calculations based on the best estimate of possible fracture reduction by calcium supplements in older women (perhaps 12%), together with the new data on vascular events, suggest that the risks of calcium supplements alone could possibly exceed the benefits. These findings clearly need to be confirmed, and it would be premature to abandon calcium supplements in groups likely to have real dietary inadequacy.

Furthermore, the results do not necessarily apply to patients taking other medications for osteoporosis such as a bisphosphonate (see Chapter 19), which may themselves be protective against vascular calcification and vascular events.

A reasonable position to take, while further research is being done on the risks and benefits of calcium supplements, may be that if a daily calcium supplement is required, in addition to the patient's diet, 1000 mg of elemental calcium is probably sufficient for all patients and it should be taken in divided doses, two or three times daily, to minimize increases in the blood calcium level.

Risk of kidney stones

There is a small increase in the risk of kidney stones from calcium supplements, something that is particularly relevant to patients with a past history of calcium-containing kidney stones. Most calcium kidney stones consist of calcium oxalate. If calcium supplements are given with meals, the food binds the oxalate so that less is absorbed (and therefore less is excreted in the urine), and this may help to offset any increase in stone risk. If calcium supplements are given to a patient with a history of calcium-containing kidney stones, once the patient has stabilized on the supplement (say after two weeks), the patient's urine calcium should be measured (usually in a 24-hour urine collection), to ensure that it is not increased above normal, which is a clear risk factor for more stones. In that case, the calcium supplement should be reduced, or a medication added that specifically lowers the urinary output of calcium, such as a thiazide diuretic (type of "water pill") or related drug (chlorthalidone or indapamide). Because thiazide diuretics such as hydrochlorothiazide uniquely reduce calcium losses into the urine, this family of drugs has been studied to determine if they might be effective as a treatment for osteoporosis. They may help a little, but any effects are small.

Because citrate in the urine inhibits stone formation, it has been suggested that calcium citrate might be preferable to other calcium supplements in blunting the risk of stone formation, though this has not been proved in clinical trials.

The fate of dietary calcium

An adult eating a normal diet containing a total of about 1000 mg of elemental calcium per day absorbs only about 20%, or 200 mg,

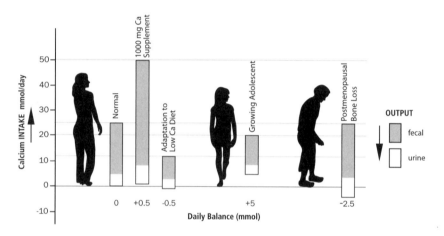

Figure 10: Overall calcium balance in various clinical situations

The total intake of calcium (diet plus supplements) is measured upwards from the zero line and ranges from 12.5 to 50 mmol in the various circumstances. Note that 1 mmol calcium equals 40 mg, hence 12.5 mmol equals 500 mg and 50 mmol equals 2000 mg. The loss of calcium in the feces is shown in grey and the loss in urine in white. The difference between the sum of these losses and the intake represents the daily overall balance. In a normal individual, overall balance is zero. When intake is increased, e.g. with a calcium supplement, there is initial transient positive balance, but rapid adaptation occurs, with a return almost to zero balance, as shown. Similarly adaptation can occur with a low intake, again with a close to zero balance, as shown. The growing adolescent is in strongly positive overall balance (growing bones). The patient with untreated postmenopausal osteoporosis (losing bone) is in significant negative overall calcium balance, despite a normal dietary calcium intake.

from the gut into the blood stream. The remaining 80% is lost in the feces. Possible fates for the absorbed calcium include being deposited in the bone (if net bone formation is occurring) or being excreted by the kidneys into the urine. If net bone formation is zero (as much bone is being broken down as is being built up), approximately 200 mg of calcium will be excreted daily in the urine. If there is significant bone breakdown (e.g. rapidly developing osteoporosis) the daily calcium excretion will exceed the amount absorbed from the gut, whereas if there is significant net bone formation (as in the growing child), urinary calcium will be less than the amount absorbed.

Calcium adaptation

Long ago, researchers documented an interesting phenomenon regarding the absorption of dietary calcium which they called "calcium adaptation". It was noted that normal people adjust their intestinal calcium absorption according to their dietary calcium intake. When placed on a low calcium intake, a larger fraction of the dietary calcium is absorbed, whereas increases in dietary calcium reduced the efficiency of absorption (see Figure 10). This normal adaptation is now known to involve vitamin D. It would be anticipated that this adaptation might limit the benefits to be gained from dietary calcium supplements, though it may also help to reduce the frequency of kidney stones in users of calcium supplements. It may also explain why populations consuming calcium intakes well below recommended levels do not necessarily have a high incidence of osteoporosis. Adaptation is an important process in younger individuals; it is possible that it becomes less efficient with increasing age.

Some other dietary constituents have effects on calcium

Dietary protein, salt and perhaps caffeine may cause excessive loss of calcium into the urine, which may not be offset by increased absorption of calcium from the diet. Such a process, continued over a long period of time, might result in loss of calcium from the bone and perhaps contribute to the development of osteoporosis.

Idiopathic hypercalciuria

There are also individuals in the population who habitually excrete greater than normal amounts of calcium in the urine. This condition is called idiopathic hypercalciuria. Patients with this problem most often come to light as a result of symptoms resulting from the formation of kidney stones. The reason for the increased urinary calcium excretion is not fully understood. The calcium concentration in the blood is normal but calcium absorption from food is usually greater than normal. In addition to causing kidney stones, hypercalciuria is sometimes found in patients with osteoporosis. Treatment with drugs that lower urinary calcium excretion reduces the risk of stone recurrence, and may be of some benefit for the associated osteoporosis.

CHAPTER THIRTEEN

Parathyroid hormone (PTH)

THE MECHANISM THROUGH WHICH the calcium level in the blood (serum calcium level) is so exquisitely regulated is well understood and is mainly the work of the parathyroid glands. Each person normally has four such glands, two on either side of the neck, each about the size of a lentil. The parathyroid glands secrete a hormone called parathyroid hormone (PTH) into the bloodstream.

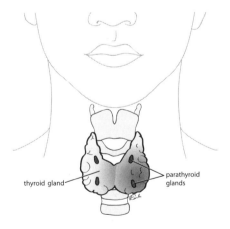

Figure 11: The normal parathyroid glands
The four normal parathyroid glands lie in the front of the neck, in contact with the thyroid gland.

Until quite recently, it was not understood how the parathyroid glands monitor and respond to changes in the serum calcium level. About a decade ago, researchers showed that the cells of the parathyroid glands have calcium sensors on their surfaces, by means of which they continuously monitor the free calcium ion level in the blood serum. This calcium sensing receptor (CaSR) is a protein molecule, which presumably undergoes changes in its shape (conformation) in response to changing serum calcium ion concentrations, giving rise to a signal in the parathyroid cell telling it to increase or decrease its secretion of parathyroid hormone (PTH) into the blood stream.

PTH is a protein hormone with effects on bone, kidney and other organs. There is normally a low baseline level of PTH secretion, and a low but measurable concentration of PTH in the blood. In normal individuals, the secretion of PTH is shut off if the blood calcium concentration rises, even minimally, whereas a fall in the calcium concentration triggers an increase in PTH secretion. The effect of the hormone is to raise the blood calcium level through three principal actions:

1. On the bone, to stimulate osteoclasts to release more calcium into the blood;
2. On the kidney, to reduce calcium losses into the urine;
3. On the intestine, to (indirectly) increase the absorption of calcium from the diet.

When the calcium concentration returns to its normal range, the output of PTH again decreases to its low baseline level.

Even in severe osteoporosis, the quantity of calcium available in the bones is so huge, relative to the small amount of calcium in the blood, that under the influence of PTH it can be drawn upon almost indefinitely for the maintenance of the normal serum calcium level. Thus the serum calcium level remains normal in osteoporosis, and is of no value as an indicator of the existence or severity of osteoporosis. Rather, an abnormal serum calcium level usually indicates a separate problem with the parathyroid glands or parathyroid hormone.

Thus, during a long period of severe dietary calcium deprivation, calcium derived from the bone mineral (rather than the diet) is utilized to maintain the normal calcium concentration in the blood. Over time, this can cause significant leaching of calcium from the bones, and hence can contribute to the development of osteoporosis.

Later on in this book, thoughtful readers will understandably be confused by the paradox that PTH is now being used to treat osteoporosis, despite the fact that its usual physiological effect is to promote the release of calcium from bone! Suffice it to say that (for reasons that are still incompletely understood) intermittent subcutaneous injections of PTH once daily, as used in the treatment of osteoporosis, have quite a different effect on bone from the more stable, lower level of PTH that is present under normal circumstances. Rather than causing net loss of calcium from bone, daily PTH injections, over time, cause increased accumulation of calcium in the bone, with an increase in bone mineral density, and reversal of osteoporosis.

Primary hyperparathyroidism (PHP)

This is a condition in which one or more of the parathyroid glands becomes enlarged and secretes inappropriately large amounts of parathyroid hormone. The abnormal glands are almost always benign (not cancerous). The hallmark of this condition is an increased calcium level in the blood – hypercalcemia. If PTH is also increased, the diagnosis is virtually certain since under normal circumstances an elevated calcium level would cause the parathyroid glands to reduce their level of PTH secretion. In primary hyperparathyroidism the excretion of calcium in the urine is usually increased, and this is probably the main reason why kidney stones occur in primary hyperparathyroidism.

The most common clinical problems in primary hyperparathyroidism are kidney stones (in about 5% of patients) and bone disease. The bone disease can take a different form from osteoporosis, in which single or multiple bone cysts occur (so-called osteitis fibrosa cystica), but for unclear reasons that condition is becoming very rare in high-income countries. Much more often the bones are normal, or the bone mineral density shows a reduction which may be generalized, or may preferentially affect cortical bone, for example in the forearm.

Nowadays most patients with primary hyperparathyroidism are diagnosed as a result of a routine testing of the blood calcium level. If patients have no symptoms and the calcium level in the blood is only modestly elevated, they are usually not sent for surgical treatment, but rather undergo regular check-up to exclude important complications that might indicate a need for surgery. However, severe hypercalcemia, kidney stones or a significantly reduced bone mineral density would all be regarded as indications for referral to a surgeon for removal of the abnormal parathyroid gland(s).

Identifying which parathyroid gland is responsible for primary hyperparathyroidism can sometimes be a challenge. Various tests are used, including nuclear medicine scans, ultrasound, etc. If it is thought that a single gland is the problem, and it has been located before surgery, it can be removed with a small operation. However, if the offending gland has not been localized before surgery it is necessary for the surgeon to identify all four glands—a significantly larger operation—and to remove any that are abnormal. Sometimes all four glands are enlarged in which case most of the glandular tissue (3½ glands) may need to be removed.

After surgical removal of the offending gland(s), kidney stone formation greatly decreases, and the bone mineral density usually shows a rapid improvement. Non-surgical treatments for primary hyperparathyroidism have not been satisfactory in the past, but there is interest in the possible use of "calcimimetic" drugs (drugs that mimic calcium), which interact with the calcium receptor on the parathyroid cells to decrease parathyroid hormone production, in patients who are not suitable candidates for surgery.

Cancer-related hypercalcemia

The two most common causes of a high calcium level in the blood (known as hypercalcemia) are parathyroid gland overactivity (primary hyperparathyroidism) and cancers.

Hypercalcemia has long been noted in cancer patients (lung, breast, kidney) but no one really understood why it happened. Sometimes these cancers will spread to the skeleton, and in the past it was thought that this might be the reason; the cancer cells were causing bone resorption. Another long-standing theory was that these cancers were producing and secreting parathyroid hormone, in the same way that cancers can secrete other hormones. This may seem like a wildly improbable scenario, until it is appreciated that all of the cells in the body contain the genetic code required to produce any human protein.

With increasingly refined parathyroid hormone assays, however, it became clear that it was not parathyroid hormone (PTH) that these cancers were producing, but a related protein hormone now known as PTH-related Peptide (PTHrP) which causes most cancer-related hypercalcemia. The role of PTHrP in health is not fully understood, but it is thought to be particularly important in regulating calcium in the fetus and during lactation in the mother. Because PTHrP shares most of the actions of PTH, it is being studied as another possible treatment for osteoporosis.

CHAPTER FOURTEEN

Calcitonin

CALCITONIN, LIKE PARATHYROID HORMONE (PTH), is a protein hormone. It is produced by special cells of the thyroid gland (C cells). Its actions oppose those of PTH and so calcitonin *lowers* the concentration of calcium in the blood. It was discovered by the late Dr. Harold Copp, then the Professor of Physiology at the University of British Columbia in Vancouver. Calcitonin may have been more important at earlier stages of evolution, for example in fish, than it is in mammals. Calcitonin lowers the blood calcium level by inhibiting osteoclasts. It does not appear to be very important in normal human physiology, since the thyroid gland can be removed without significant adverse effects on calcium metabolism. In addition to its effects on calcium and bone, calcitonin has a modest pain-relieving (analgesic) action, probably through direct effects on the brain.

Calcitonin is produced by certain thyroid tumors, in which measurement of calcitonin levels in the blood provide a useful marker of tumor activity. Because it inhibits osteoclasts, it was anticipated that calcitonin would be useful in the treatment of osteoporosis. It was found to be effective, but had to be given by injection, or more recently by nasal spray. It has largely been replaced as treatment by the more potent and more convenient bisphosphonates, but nasal calcitonin may still have a place in the acute treatment of patients with severe pain after a vertebral fracture. However, unless significant benefit is seen within two weeks, it should be replaced with alternative therapies.

Calcitonin is discussed further in Chapter 21.

CHAPTER FIFTEEN

Vitamin D

VITAMIN D IS AN IMPORTANT REGULATOR of calcium in the body. Its most important action is to increase the absorption of calcium from food in the intestine into the bloodstream.

Vitamin D produced in the skin

Most vitamins are derived only from the diet, and deficiency arises when the diet is inadequate, or when absorption of the vitamin from the food is reduced, for example due to intestinal disease. For vitamin D, however, the situation is a little more complicated. Vitamin D is not only derived from food, but is also made *in the skin* in response to exposure to sunlight (ultraviolet light). This is the primary source of vitamin D in nature. It is actually vitamin D3 that is produced in the skin.

It is suggested that exposure of the arms and legs, around midday, for five to thirty minutes twice weekly (depending on season and latitude) can produce sufficient vitamin D for the body's needs. Sunscreen and skin pigmentation reduce vitamin D production in the skin, and production of vitamin D is less efficient in the elderly. Many individuals do not achieve adequate skin production of vitamin D year round, and are therefore dependent upon additional vitamin D from the diet, especially in winter time and at more northern latitudes.

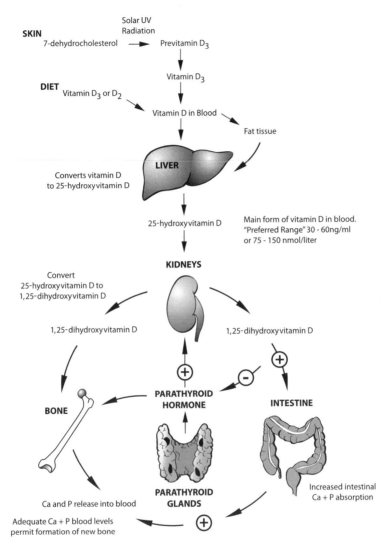

Figure 12: Vitamin D; sources, metabolism and actions in the body
Vitamin D originating from solar ultraviolet irradiation of the skin, or from the diet, undergoes successive changes in the liver and the kidneys to form its final active product, 1,25-dihydroxyvitamin D (1,25(OH)$_2$D). 1,25(OH)$_2$D acts on the intestine to promote calcium absorption and on the bone, in concert with parathyroid hormone (PTH), to promote calcium release into the blood. Ultimately all of these actions of vitamin D help to maintain the normal calcium level in the blood. 1,25(OH)$_2$D also acts directly on the parathyroid glands to reduce PTH release. Based on Holick MF, Vitamin D Deficiency, New England Journal of Medicine, 2007, 357, 266-281.

Vitamin D from the diet

The main dietary sources of vitamin D are fish oils and fortified foods. Vitamin D2 and D3 are slightly different chemical forms of vitamin D that were assumed to be equally effective. However, it has recently been shown that vitamin D2 has a much shorter half-life in the body than vitamin D3, and is therefore significantly less effective (at a given dose) in humans than vitamin D3. Vitamin D3 is usually the form which is added to fortified foods, and present in most vitamin D supplements in Canada. Formerly vitamin D supplements consisted of vitamin D2.

Activation of vitamin D in the liver and kidneys

In order for vitamin D3 or D2 to be effective, they must undergo sequential chemical change in the liver, and subsequently in the kidney. The liver converts vitamin D into 25-hydroxyvitamin D, also called 25(OH)D. The blood level of 25(OH)D is the best available index of vitamin D nutritional status, and is easily measured in the laboratory.

25(OH)D is further converted to $1,25(OH)_2D$ (1,25-dihydroxyvitamin D) in the kidneys. The blood level of $1,25(OH)_2D$ is approximately 1,000 times lower than that of 25(OH)D, but it is this $1,25(OH)_2D$ that is the active form responsible for the biological effects of vitamin D on the intestine and bone. The level of $1,25(OH)_2D$ in the blood can also be measured in the laboratory, but it is a more difficult and expensive test than 25(OH)D, and is not a useful index of vitamin D nutrition.

Actions of vitamin D

There are vitamin D receptors in the cells lining the inner surface of the small intestine, with which $1,25(OH)_2D$ combines to initiate the biological effects, particularly increased absorption of calcium and phosphate from the food. There are also vitamin D receptors in the cells of many other organs, including bone and kidney.

A major determinant of the conversion of 25(OH)D to $1,25(OH)_2D$ in the kidneys is parathyroid hormone (PTH). In conditions in which PTH levels are higher, more $1,25(OH)_2D$ is produced and by this mechanism more of the body's vitamin D is "activated". This is the indirect mechanism through which PTH enhances the intestinal absorption of calcium. In kidney disease, especially kidney failure, the production of $1,25(OH)_2D$ from $25(OH)D$ in the kidneys is inadequate, leading to poor calcium absorption from the food. Many such patients require treatment with $1,25(OH)_2D$.

As noted, the most important action of $1,25(OH)_2D$ is to promote the absorption of calcium from food in the intestine. Significant vitamin D deficiency would be expected to reduce calcium absorption from the diet, and therefore to reduce the excretion of calcium in the urine. While vitamin D deficiency is best identified by measuring the $25(OH)D$ level in the blood, the demonstration of a very low urinary calcium, though much less specific, may be a useful and inexpensive screening test for vitamin D deficiency.

How much vitamin D do we need?

Like the issue of who needs calcium supplements, and how much, controversy surrounds the subject of vitamin D requirements, the need for supplements, and the amounts needed. In part, this results from a lack of consensus on how "optimal" vitamin D nutrition should be defined. One possible way would be measurement of $25(OH)D$ levels, but that requires agreement on what is an optimal level. Another possibility is to measure PTH levels, on the assumption that PTH will begin to rise as vitamin D becomes deficient. However, many other factors can influence PTH levels.

As was suggested for calcium supplements, it may be best to try to target those sections of the population in whom sun exposure and vitamin D nutrition are most likely to be inadequate, rather than giving large supplements of vitamin D indiscriminately to everyone. This would include the elderly, especially those living alone or institutionalized, as well as people living in countries where sunshine is scarce, where exposure of the skin to sunlight is minimized (e.g. by wearing clothing that leaves little skin exposed) and/or where foods are not supplemented with vitamin D.

Notwithstanding the large number of studies performed in the past, further studies are needed to define precisely when and how vitamin D supplements should be used in osteoporosis. Such studies should include measurements of vitamin D levels in the blood, should take account of calcium intakes, and should recognize the differences in the biological efficacy of vitamin D2 versus vitamin D3.

Until recently, 400–800 units per day of vitamin D were considered to be adequate, in the absence of disease of the intestine compromising vitamin D absorption, or of drugs that interfere with vitamin D metabolism such as anticonvulsants. Many experts are now recommending much higher doses to prevent vitamin D deficiency, for example 1,000–2,000 units per day or 100,000 units once every two months. Vitamin D does not need to be administered frequently because large doses are retained for two months in the tissues, including fat. The ability to give infrequent large doses of vitamin D may significantly improve patient adherence, in comparison with calcium, which should be given at least once every day. Elderly individuals may need 800–1,600 units of vitamin D per day.

As far as is known, there is little or no down-side to taking vitamin D supplements in the recommended doses, in order to achieve optimal serum 25(OH)D levels of 75 nmol/L (30 ng/ml). It is estimated that, for every increase in the daily dose of vitamin D supplement of 100 units, the average increase in the 25(OH)D level is about 2.5 nmol/L (1 ng/ml). Thus, a patient with a 25(OH)D level of 50 nmol/L (20 ng/ml) is likely to require an additional 1,000 units of vitamin D per day to achieve a 25(OH)D level of 75 nmol/L (30 ng/ml). There may be some increase in the risk of calcium stone formation, but this has not been well documented. Vitamin D intoxication occurs when the 25(OH)D level is 375 nmol/L (150 ng/ml) or greater, so there is a considerable margin of safety. Vitamin D intoxication usually results from excessive consumption of vitamin D supplements. It causes a rise in the calcium level in the urine and the blood, which can be associated with serious problems including kidney failure.

There is great current interest in actions of vitamin D other than the traditional ones on bone and mineral metabolism. It is being used in the treatment of some forms of leukemia and psoriasis. There is also some evidence that vitamin D may help to prevent colorectal, and possibly breast and prostate cancers. In addition, vitamin D also has direct effects on muscle, improving muscle strength, which may be relevant in osteoporosis as it may help to reduce the risk of falls.

Vitamin D deficiency, as would be expected, is a particular problem in winter time in northern latitudes. Recently it has been suggested that relative vitamin D deficiency may contribute to diseases that are more common at higher latitudes, such as multiple sclerosis.

We shall return to the use of vitamin D supplements in the prevention and treatment of osteoporosis in Chapter 16.

| **Osteoporosis prevention and treatment**

Preventing osteoporosis

Physical activity with avoidance of falls, supplements (calcium and vitamin D) and diet

THE COMBINATION OF "LIFESTYLE" MEASURES comprising an optimal dietary intake of calcium and vitamin D and an appropriate exercise program has traditionally underpinned most osteoporosis prevention or treatment regimens. Avoidance of smoking and excess alcohol intake, which also promote osteoporosis, are other good things to do.

The objective of osteoporosis preventative measures is to try to slow the decline in bone mineral density that usually occurs with aging. As previously noted, bone mineral density is a predictor of fracture, albeit an imperfect one, but it is statistically better than is blood pressure as an indicator for stroke.

Individuals who should follow prudent "lifestyle" measures include:

1. Normal people with no indication for DXA testing.
2. People whose bone mineral density is in the normal or low fracture risk range (formerly often called osteopenic), who have no specific indications for drug treatment for osteoporosis.
3. People requiring active treatment for established osteoporosis, in whom other osteoporosis medications will usually be given as well.

Physical activity and avoidance of falls

Immobilization or prolonged bed rest are well recognized to worsen osteoporosis. Weightlessness also leads to rapid bone loss and may be an important issue on long space flights in the future.

Regular weight bearing exercise is recommended for the prevention and treatment of osteoporosis, and has been shown to help maintain or even produce a modest increase in bone mineral density. Walking for 90 to 280 minutes per week produced a small improvement in spinal bone mineral density, but no change at the femur (thigh bone). In school children regular exercise has been shown to improve bone mass, but has to be continued, otherwise the benefit is lost. There are no large trials establishing whether these interventions reduce the fracture risk.

Falls are a stronger risk factor for hip fracture than a decrease in bone mineral density, and so preventing falls is an important part of preventing fractures. The practical question, however, is whether we have effective means to prevent falls. A number of approaches have been tried, including strength and balance training, reducing the dose and frequency of psychotropic drugs (drugs used for depression/anxiety), calcium and vitamin D supplements (vitamin D may help muscle strength), and assessment and modification of home hazards.

Some earlier studies were positive regarding the usefulness of falls prevention programs, to the extent that the UK's National Health Service "Framework for Older People" required the establishment of falls prevention programs. Unfortunately, more recent examination of available data has been inconclusive with regard to whether these programs show a benefit.

Another approach is the use of hip protectors to pad the hip in the event of a fall. These were originally reported to reduce hip fractures, but more recent studies have shown inconsistent results, and patient adherence tends to be poor. Most patients simply don't want to wear the padded undergarments. They may be most effective in institutionalized elderly patients.

Calcium and vitamin D intake
Calcium intake

This has been discussed in detail in Chapter 2, including reference to some recent concerns about a possible association of vascular events (such as heart attacks) with long-term calcium supplements. Individuals at all stages of their lives have been encouraged to achieve "adequate" calcium intakes, either through diet alone, or with the addition of calcium supplements. A problem has been the difficulty in agreeing what constitutes an "adequate" intake of calcium.

It is believed that ingested calcium supplements can enhance peak bone mass and slow the decline in bone mineral density with aging. It is likely, however, that studies showing a beneficial effect of calcium supplements on bone mineral density included substantial numbers of individuals who were previously taking low calcium intakes, including elderly and institutionalized people, and those who avoid dairy products, so the studies might not represent what would happen to more typical people taking supplements.

In an analysis of multiple studies, calcium supplementation caused a 1.5–2% improvement in bone mineral density at spine, hip and wrist, and there was no difference between dairy sources of calcium and calcium supplements. In older men and women a calcium intake of 1000 mg per day has been shown to lower the bone remodeling rate and to increase bone mineral density over the first 12–18 months. *(see Figure 13 on next page)*

The approximate requirement for calcium supplementation can be calculated by estimating the elemental calcium content of an individual's diet and determining if this is less than the recommended daily intake. There is no evidence that increasing calcium intake above the recommended daily intake provides any additional benefit. Calcium supplementation may be achieved either by increasing calcium-containing foods (usually dairy products) or with calcium supplements. There is no evidence to support the notion that calcium from dairy products is any better than calcium from supplements. In choosing a calcium supplement, it is important to appreciate that the quantities referred to above relate to elemental calcium.

The recent concerns regarding vascular complications arising from calcium supplements, as well as the more recent study which failed to confirm an association between coronary calcification and calcium supplements underline the need to conduct more research on the risk:benefit ratio for calcium supplements, perhaps especially when used alone, and in older women. In the meantime,

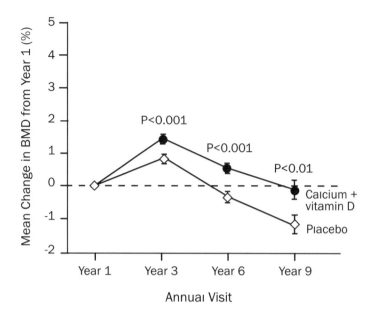

Figure 13: Effect of calcium (1000 mg) plus vitamin D (400 units) supplementation compared with placebo over a nine year period in 36,000 healthy post-menopausal women

There was no significant reduction in hip fractures in the treated group compared with placebo, nor were significant differences observed in bone mineral density at the spine. In this study, however, (as shown), a small but significant 1% improvement in bone mineral density was observed at the hip in the calcium and vitamin D group compared with placebo. This study, like many others, suggests that the benefits from calcium and vitamin D supplementation may be quite small in healthy women. They are likely to be greater in individuals with pre-existing deficiencies of calcium or vitamin D. From Jackson RD et al., Calcium plus vitamin D supplementation and the risk of fractures. New England Journal of Medicine, 2006, 354, 669-83.

it would seem prudent not to exceed total daily intakes (in the diet plus supplements) of 1,000 to a maximum of 1500 mg.

Furthermore, if the theory that adverse vascular effects could be related to transient increases in the calcium level in the blood following calcium dosing is correct, it would seem wise to avoid taking large single doses of calcium. It has generally been recommended that not more than 500 mg (as elemental calcium) be taken at once. Perhaps this should be reduced, for example to a maximum of 300 mg of supplemental calcium at a time, which would still allow for three daily doses of 300 mg with main meals, or a maximum total daily calcium supplement of 900–1000 mg, sufficient even for patients taking very little calcium in their diet. It is of interest that, in the recent study suggesting an adverse effect of calcium supplements, calcium was prescribed in a dose of 400 mg in the morning and 600 mg with the evening meal, in the form of calcium citrate, which may be a rather rapidly absorbed form of calcium supplement.

Excessive intakes of foods that may increase calcium requirements, such as salt and meat protein, should be avoided, as should excess alcohol (three or more drinks per day). As noted elsewhere, calcium supplements may slightly increase the risk of forming calcium containing kidney stones.

There is no good evidence of important differences between various calcium supplements. Calcium carbonate is the cheapest, and is well absorbed if taken with food. Calcium citrate might be a preferable supplement in the patient with a history of kidney stones. Supplements containing magnesium (or other minerals) are not generally required unless there are other medical problems that could increase the need for magnesium. Contrary to what is sometimes stated in the complementary or alternative medicine literature, magnesium is not required to facilitate calcium absorption. A magnesium-containing calcium supplement may be useful, however, to counteract the slightly constipating effects of calcium experienced by some people.

Vitamin D

In Chapter 15, detailed consideration was given to vitamin D, and particularly to the current controversy regarding human vitamin D requirements. As in the case of calcium, efforts to increase vitamin D intakes should particularly target those populations most at risk for vitamin D deficiency—the old and the institutionalized, those who get little ultraviolet skin exposure and those on inadequate diets or with intestinal disease.

Whereas some studies have failed to show an effect of vitamin D supplements (in conventional doses of 400 to 800 units per day) on fracture risk, others have suggested that a 25(OH)D level of about 75 nmol/L (30 ng/ml) is required to show benefit. The intakes of vitamin D recently recommended by some authorities are those required to achieve serum 25(OH)D levels of 75–80 nmol/L (30–32 ng/ml). These doses are higher than previously recommended. Some authorities are now recommending 1,000 to 2,000 units per day for the patient with osteoporosis.

Rather than daily vitamin D dosing, the vitamin can be given in large infrequent doses by mouth or by injection. Some patients adhere to a once monthly regime better than to daily pills. A regime of 50,000 units once monthly by mouth achieved the desired 25(OH) D level in the blood in most patients after a few months.

At the present time, a prudent total daily intake of vitamin D is around 1,000 units. In some countries, vitamin D derivatives such as 1,25(OH)$_2$D or 1 alpha hydroxy D (which is converted in the body to 1,25(OH)$_2$D) are used for the treatment of osteoporosis. There is no convincing evidence that they are more effective than traditional vitamin D, and furthermore, they carry a much greater risk of causing vitamin D intoxication. Their use in the treatment of osteoporosis is therefore not recommended.

In order to ensure that patients with osteoporosis take their vitamin D, some pharmaceutical companies have been adding vitamin D to their bisphosphonate medications so that patients take both together. Vitamin D is also included in some calcium supplements.

Evidence for the efficacy of "adequate calcium and vitamin D" intakes

Raising the 25(OH) D levels has been shown to increase intestinal calcium absorption and to reduce the rate of bone loss. Vitamin D supplements also improve muscle strength and reduce falls. There is reasonable evidence that calcium and vitamin D supplements, particularly in individuals with dietary deficiency, are beneficial. The evidence that calcium and vitamin D supplements actually decrease fractures is somewhat inconsistent. However, a recent review concluded that 1200 mg calcium plus at least 800 units of vitamin D daily reduced fractures by 12% in men and women over age 50.

In studies of the active drug treatments to be considered later, both the treatment group and the placebo group have generally been given calcium and vitamin D supplements (usually in fairly low doses) in order to ensure that any differences attributable to the drug could not be due to unintended differences in calcium or vitamin D intakes between groups. The recent concern about possible vascular risks of calcium supplements when used as sole treatment for osteoporosis in older women may or may not be relevant to other patient groups including those on concurrent active drug treatment such as a bisphosphonate. There is an urgent need for more studies of the risk:benefit ratio of calcium and vitamin D supplements.

There are many misconceptions about the relationship between dietary calcium and vitamin D and osteoporosis. Although there is evidence from many studies that, under certain circumstances, supplements of calcium and vitamin D can slightly improve bone mineral density and can reduce fracture risk, the effects are comparatively small. It is also a common misconception that an individual who has consistently taken an adequate intake of calcium and vitamin D and been reasonably physically active is protected from osteoporosis. Alas, that is not the case. Heredity is probably a very much more important determinant of whether an individual will get osteoporosis than are calcium and vitamin D intakes and/or exercise. Nonetheless, it appears prudent, in the present state of knowledge, to avoid dietary insufficiency of calcium and vitamin D, but the time may have come to move away from the indiscriminate use of large calcium supplements, as discussed above.

Kidney stones

One of the consequences of increasing calcium (and vitamin D) intake may be an increase in the urinary output of calcium, which is a risk factor for calcium stones. However, it is not currently recommended that the dietary calcium intake should be restricted below normal in patients with recurrent calcium stones, because it has been shown that this does not reduce their risk of stones, and may lower bone mineral density if continued for long periods of time. Rather, a normal calcium intake is recommended.

Studies on the impact of calcium supplements on calcium stones have given conflicting results, but it appears that calcium supplements taken with food may be less likely to increase the risk of stones than calcium supplements taken between meals, perhaps because calcium ingested with meals decreases oxalate absorption from the food, helping to reduce the urine saturation with calcium oxalate, the main constituent of most kidney stones.

Osteoporosis patients with a history of calcium-containing kidney stones should be given the recommended vitamin D and calcium (taken with food) intakes, and their urinary calcium should then be monitored after a few weeks. If the urinary calcium is greater than normal, the supplements can be cut back, or alternatively the high urinary calcium can be reduced with a thiazide diuretic or related drug such as chlorthalidone or indapamide.

Diet

It is recognized that the elderly, particularly those who are institutionalized, are at risk for dietary protein deficiency, which can contribute to muscle weakness and falls, and to delayed recovery from fractures. To avoid protein deficiency, they should be encouraged to consume a diet containing at least 1 gram of protein per kg body weight.

While protein deficiency is undesirable, it is possible that high protein intake, especially meat protein, may also be bad for osteoporosis. The increased consumption of protein, particularly animal protein, increases the generation of acid (mainly from sulfur-containing amino acids), which has to be excreted by the kidneys. Acid may promote calcium loss from the bone, both by a direct action on the bone mineral, and by an effect on the kidney to increase calcium loss into the urine. The administration of an alkali, such as potassium citrate, in a sufficient amount to neutralize the acid generated from dietary protein counteracts both the increased acid excretion and the increased urinary calcium loss that otherwise accompany a high protein diet.

Meat protein intake has increased in high income countries as osteoporosis has also increased. That does not prove that meat consumption causes osteoporosis, but it has generated the very interesting idea, supported by some recent data, that a low dose of an alkali such as potassium citrate, taken continuously, might help to reduce the risk of developing osteoporosis. Presumably a substantial decrease in meat protein intake would be similarly effective. However, the protein intake should not be too low—as noted above, an intake of at least 1 gram of protein per kg body weight is recommended.

An increase in the dietary intake of salt also increases calcium losses in the urine. These are generally offset by increased calcium absorption from the gut. However, there may be individuals in whom this compensation is incomplete, and hence avoidance of high salt intakes has been suggested.

Much more research is needed in order to develop specific recommendations regarding appropriate consumption of protein, alkali supplements, salt and caffeine in persons with osteoporosis, or concerned about developing it.

CHAPTER SEVENTEEN

Hormone replacement therapy in postmenopausal women

USUAL REPLACEMENT DOSES OF FEMALE HORMONES (e.g. 0.625 mg of premarin and 2.5 mg of provera daily or equivalent doses of other preparations), if given from the first symptoms of menopause ("perimenopause", which precedes the cessation of menstruation) through menopause, prevent or at least lessen the phase of rapid bone loss that normally accompanies the "estrogen deficiency" of the immediate post menopause. This type of hormone replacement therapy (HRT) has been used to alleviate menopausal symptoms, but was also a cornerstone of osteoporosis prevention and treatment until recent years.

It has been known for many years that long-term estrogen use increases the risk of breast and uterine cancer, though the use of progesterone along with the estrogen minimized or counteracted the risk of uterine cancer. Uterine cancer is not an issue in patients who have had a hysterectomy, and who can take estrogen alone.

The important question with regard to osteoporosis patients is whether the benefits of "hormone replacement" outweigh the risks. Long-term hormone replacement, particularly estrogen, had been considered to decrease the risk of degenerative vascular disease, with its associated heart attacks and strokes. However, large recent studies have shown that estrogen does not confer protection against heart attacks and strokes; indeed the risk is increased with estrogen/progesterone. Estrogen also increases the risk of blood clots and pulmonary embolism. The accumulation of better long-term data showed that the risk of breast cancer (with estrogen/progesterone combinations) is increased, and it is now generally accepted that the risks of long-term hormone replacement therapy exceed the benefits when used in the traditional manner for the prevention or treatment of osteoporosis. Fortunately, this realization more or less coincided with the availability of alternative drugs for the treatment of osteoporosis.

Although the routine use of hormone replacement therapy for osteoporosis has essentially ceased, some experts still feel there may be a place for lower dose estrogen in the management of osteoporosis.

Large studies have shown that bone mineral density increases and fractures decrease during and after long-term estrogen treatment. As with some other treatments, the relationship between the increased bone mineral density and the decrease in fractures is not simple. Less than 20% of the fracture reduction can be accounted for by the increase in bone mineral density. Also the fracture reduction appears early, before any significant change is seen in bone mineral density. It is likely that the rapid estrogen-induced decrease in bone remodeling itself reduces fracture risk, possibly by reducing trabecular perforation by osteoclasts in bone remodeling units. Moreover, estrogen may have osteoblast-stimulating properties itself.

There is some evidence that doses of estrogen lower than those used in conventional hormone replacement therapy may nonetheless produce some reduction of bone remodeling but with lower risk—for example, as little as 0.14 mg of estradiol daily, transdermally (via the skin patch). Further studies of this low dose estrogen strategy are required to determine its risk:benefit ratio, but meanwhile it is recommended that estrogens be used only short-term, and only for the relief of menopausal symptoms, not osteoporosis.

Discontinuation of estrogen is followed by a decline in bone mineral density and an increase in fracture risk, but it is not clear whether this is as rapid as that which follows the natural menopause.

CHAPTER EIGHTEEN

The influence of genetics

HEREDITY IS BELIEVED TO BE RESPONSIBLE for between 50 and 85% of the variance in bone mass. Stated differently, genes are a more important determinant of whether an individual develops primary osteoporosis than all other factors combined. Studies of identical twins dating back many years showed that bone mineral density is more alike in identical than non-identical twins, confirming the importance of heredity. The significance of a history of osteoporotic fractures in close blood relatives has been confirmed in large population studies.

Naturally, with the sequencing of the human genome in hand, there is currently great interest in trying to identify which particular genes are responsible for the inheritance of bone mineral density and bone strength. In recent large studies from the Icelandic population, many of whom have had their genome sequenced, bone mineral density and fractures were found to be linked with multiple genetic loci, including regions in close proximity to genes for RANKL and osteoprotegerin (see Appendix I) and the estrogen receptor 1. Earlier studies had suggested a role for other genes in influencing bone mineral density, including the gene for the vitamin D receptor and one of the collagen genes but these were not confirmed in the Icelandic study. More recently the number of genetic sites (loci) associated with bone density has increased to 13, and it is likely to go on increasing. In other words, like many other common diseases, osteoporosis is the result of the interaction of many genes.

It is also possible that genes could affect bone size and geometry, and therefore fracture risk, independently of the bone mineral density. At the present time, genetic testing is not useful in determining fracture risk, or in the clinical management of idiopathic osteoporosis.

Drug treatments for osteoporosis

CHAPTER NINETEEN

Bisphosphonates

When proper lifestyle, diet and supplements are not enough

IN THE PATIENT WITH A FRAGILITY FRACTURE and/or a high fracture risk, optimal diet, supplements, and exercise are recommended, but are insufficient on their own to restore a satisfactory bone mineral density or to substantially reduce fracture risk. Such patients require the addition of active drug treatment.

Medications used in the treatment of osteoporosis generally fall into one of two overall categories. They are either antiresorptive drugs or anabolic agents. Antiresorptive drugs suppress the normal process of bone turnover, while anabolic agents produce a gain of normal bone.

Considering these two categories of medications, one would naturally assume that anabolic treatment would be the treatment of choice. If the available medications were equally convenient to take, and if the cost were similar, anabolic treatment might well be the first choice in most patients. However, because the principal available anabolic treatment (parathyroid hormone or teriparatide) is extremely expensive and requires daily injections, for the moment antiresorptives (bisphosphonates), which have been shown to be very effective, are the first-line treatment for most patients.

Bisphosphonates

The bisphosphonates are a class of drugs with various actions on bone, especially antiresorptive or "anti-remodeling" effects, which can lead to an increase in bone mineral density and a reduction in fracture risk when used in the treatment of osteoporosis. They are typically the first-line treatment in osteoporosis patients who require more than lifestyle measures to reduce their fracture risk.

The history of bisphosphonates

Chemists have long known that the pyrophosphate can act as a water softener by interfering with calcium carbonate crystallization. In the 1960s, when pyrophosphate was identified in human blood and urine, scientists began to wonder if it might act as a natural water softener, inhibiting the crystallization of calcium phosphate in the body. This was supported by the recognition that an inherited disease called hypophosphatasia, in which pyrophosphate levels in the blood are increased, is characterized by a defect in the mineralization of bone.

At the time, researchers were working on ways to prevent abnormal calcification in the body. It was thought that pyrophosphate administration might help to prevent abnormal calcification, but pyrophosphate proved to be too unstable (it lost its chemical properties) when given by mouth. This led to the study of related compounds that might be suitable when taken by mouth, and specifically to the study of bisphosphonates. Bisphosphonates proved to be sufficiently stable to be administered by mouth, and to prevent abnormal mineralization.

Curiously, bisphosphonates also displayed the ability to interfere with the dissolving of apatite bone crystals during resorption, i.e. they had an antiresorptive effect. This was initially thought to be due to the physical effect of bisphosphonate incorporation into apatite crystals, but it has become clear that bisphosphonates have direct effects on osteoclasts, suppressing their activity and leading to apoptosis (cell death).

Actions of bisphosphonates

Bisphosphonates bind strongly to bone mineral (apatite). The first bisphosphonate to be used in humans was etidronate

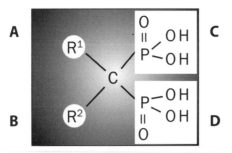

Figure 14: Chemical structure of bisphosphonate drugs
C and D are phosphonate groups, which are essential for binding to bone mineral (apatite) and for the mechanism of action on osteoclasts. A When R1 is a hydroxyl (OH) group, binding to apatite is enhanced. B The group at R2 determines potency, including binding. The investigation of compounds with different groups at R2 has resulted in new drugs with up to a 10,000 times increase in potency (zoledronate compared with etidronate). Based on Russell RGG Bisphosphonates: Mode of Action and Pharmacology. Pediatrics 2007, 119, S50-162

(Didronel). It has a hydroxyl (OH) group at the R1 position. Etidronate (Didronel) decreases mineralization, as well as decreasing osteoclastic bone resorption. It was found in the 1970s to improve bone mineral density in osteoporosis, but had to be given only intermittently (rather than continuously) in order to limit the unwanted mineralization defect.

Further research on bisphosphonates then showed that changes in the group at the R2 position greatly influenced the antiresorptive potency of the drug. In particular the inclusion of different nitrogen-containing groups at the R2 position, as in alendronate (Fosamax), risedronate (Actonel), ibandronate (Boniva) and zoledronate (these will be described) increased their antiresorptive potency as much as 10,000 times!

We now know that the non-nitrogen containing bisphosphonates such as etidronate (Didronel) and the nitrogen-containing bisphosphonates such as alendronate (Fosamax) both act as osteoclast inhibitors by virtue of direct effects on the metabolism of the osteoclast, although the mechanisms of action of these two groups of bisphosphonates are different.

As osteoclasts remove bisphosphonate-containing bone, they are exposed to uniquely high concentrations of these inhibitory drugs, and their activity slows.

Bisphosphonates accumulate in bone, and bone resorption is suppressed to a stable, lower level—it does not progressively decline with time. An interesting feature of bisphosphonates is that it is the total amount given that determines the effect, making it possible to give infrequent large doses rather than frequent small doses.

The use of bisphosphonates in treatment of osteoporosis

In osteoporosis, bisphosphonates have been a great clinical and commercial success, beginning with etidronate (Didronel) in 1990, and progressing to the latest advance, a once yearly intravenous infusion of zoledronate (Aclasta [known as Reclast in the United States]).

All of the approved bisphosphonates increase bone mineral density by decreasing resorption and reducing the number of bone remodeling units (BRUs). The increase in bone mineral density results in part from a decrease in the remodeling space, and in part from increased (secondary) mineralization of maturing BRUs. The reduction in fracture risk is partly attributable to the increase in bone mineral density, but greatly exceeds that which would be expected from the increase in bone mineral density alone. It is thought that the decrease in remodeling may reduce the frequency of resorption cavities in trabeculae, potential perforation sites or mechanical stress concentrators, leading to a reduction in trabecular fracturing. Decreased remodeling also reduces the porosity of cortical bone, which may reduce the risk of fracture. Bisphosphonates cause little positive bone balance (the addition of new bone) but there is increasing evidence that there may be some improvement in trabecular architecture.

The absorption of bisphosphonates when given by mouth is quite poor, amounting generally to less than 5% of the administered dose. Absorption is further reduced by the presence of food or medications, particularly calcium supplements, in the stomach. Bisphosphonates should therefore be taken on an empty stomach, usually after an overnight fast, and no food or medications should be taken for one hour afterwards.

Safety and potential side-effects of bisphosphonates

Since their introduction, various theoretical concerns have been voiced regarding the long-term safety of this class of drugs. These have included the possibility of impaired fracture healing, over-suppression of bone turnover with long-term use (so-called "frozen bone"), and osteonecrosis of the jaw (see below). At the present time none of these appear to represent serious concerns or reasons to avoid the use of these drugs in usual doses in the treatment of osteoporosis.

Another potential problem is esophageal inflammation/ulceration if the medication gets stuck on its way down to the stomach. Bisphosphonates should therefore not be taken by mouth in patients known to have a problem with the passage of food into the stomach (such as esophageal stricture or achalasia), and the pills should be taken with an 8oz glass of water and swallowed in an upright position, and that position should be maintained for one hour (standing, or sitting upright).

As mentioned above, there has been recent concern regarding the occurrence of osteonecrosis of the jaw in patients receiving bisphosphonates. Osteonecrosis of the jaw is an unpleasant condition in which non-healing areas of exposed bone develop in the mouth, usually near the rear upper molar teeth, often following dental extractions. However, the current consensus of opinion is that this condition is sufficiently rare in patients receiving usual doses of bisphosphonate for osteoporosis (perhaps one patient in 100,000 treated cases) that it should not be regarded as a reason not to use it. Most patients with osteonecrosis of the jaw have received high doses of intravenous bisphosphonates for complications of cancer, and many have had previous surgical procedures or radiation treatment to the jaw. Nevertheless, a patient receiving bisphosphonates should advise their dentist if surgical procedures on the jaw are contemplated even though recent reviews of this issue suggest that bisphosphonate treatment for osteoporosis should not contraindicate dental implants.

The mechanism by which bisphosphonates cause osteonecrosis of the jaw is not understood. The condition is usually associated with infection in the bone, and it has been suggested that the problem may be a failure of the mucus membrane to heal, rather than a problem with the bone itself.

A concern identified from one of the recent large zoledronate (Aclasta) studies was the development of a heart rhythm disturbance (atrial fibrillation). Subsequent analysis of other bisphosphonate databases has been inconclusive, but suggests that this could be a minor problem in some elderly patients at risk for atrial fibrillation. The mechanism of such an effect is not known. There have been a few recent reports of unusual fractures of the femur in patients on bisphosphonates, but it is not yet clear whether this is a true association.

Individual bisphosphonates

Etidronate (Didronel)

Etidronate (Didronel) differs from the more recently introduced bisphosphonates such as alendronate (Fosamax) and risedronate (Actonel) in that, when given continuously, it interferes with the mineralization of newly forming bone. It has therefore been used in an intermittent, cyclical fashion. Didronel is usually given daily for the first two weeks of each three month cycle. In Canada it is generally prescribed as "Didrocal" in a three month blister pack in which 400 mg is given daily for the first twoweeks, followed by a 500 mg calcium supplement once daily for the remainder of the three month cycle. Didronel should be taken on an empty stomach, food and other medications being deferred for 30 minutes.

In the original studies of Didronel in postmenopausal women in 1990, spinal bone mineral density increased significantly, by 8% relative to placebo after 150 weeks, and a reduction of recurrent fractures at the spine was also reported. Didronel is well tolerated, but can occasionally cause some diarrhea. It is cheaper than the other bisphosphonates. Currently its main use is in patients unable to tolerate or afford the more recent and more potent and effective bisphosphonates.

Alendronate (Fosamax)

Alendronate (Fosamax) was the first of the potent bisphosphonates (containing a nitrogen group) to undergo clinical studies in osteoporosis. In the landmark study, reported in 1995, in a daily dose of 10 mg, it increased vertebral bone mineral density by 9% and femoral neck bone mineral density by 6% compared with placebo over three years. Bone turnover, as shown by measuring bone markers in the blood or urine, decreased 50–70% in the first few weeks, and this persisted for as long as the drug was given. Among patients with vertebral fractures, alendronate (Fosamax) decreased vertebral, hip and wrist fractures over three years by about 50%.

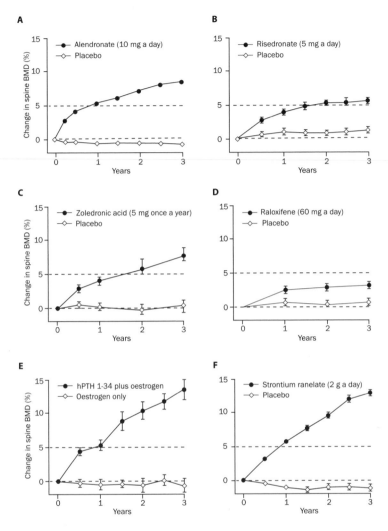

Figure 15: Effect of A – Alendronate (Fosamax), B – Risedronate (Actonel), C – Zoledronic acid, D – Raloxifene (Evista), F – Strontium ranelate compared with placebo on bone density at the spine over a three year period.
Panel E shows parathyroid hormone (PTH) as a daily injection plus estrogen compared with estrogen alone over three years in an early trial. PTH is presently only used for 18-24 month courses.

References for this figure:
Alendronate (Fosamax). Liberman UA et al., New England J Med, 1995, 333, 1437-43.
Risedronate (Actonel). Harris ST et al., JAMA, 1999, 282, 1344-52
Zoledronic acid. Black DM et al., New England J Med, 2007, 356, 1809-22
Raloxifene (Evista). Ettinger B et al., JAMA, 1999, 282, 637-645.
Strontium Ranelate. Meunier PJ et al., New England J Med, 2004, 350, 459-68.
Parathyroid hormone. Lindsay R et al., Lancet, 1997, 350, 550-555.

For the treatment of osteoporosis, alendronate (Fosamax) was initially given as 10 mg daily, but in 2000, a single 70 mg dose became available for once weekly administration, when it was shown to be as effective as the 10 mg daily dosing, at least with respect to its effects on bone markers and bone mineral density.

The ten year experience with alendronate (Fosamax) was reported in 2004 describing increases in bone mineral density averaging 13.7% at the lumbar spine, and 6.7% at the total proximal femur (hip) compared with baseline values. Markers of remodeling remained stable; there was no suggestion of an increase in fracturing. Discontinuation resulted in a gradual loss of effect in contrast to the rapid loss of the effect of estrogen, raloxifene (Evista) or parathyroid hormone when they are discontinued. Possible reasons why bone loss is slow after stopping bisphosphonates are discussed later in this chapter.

Alendronate (Fosamax) has been shown to prevent glucocorticoid-induced bone loss (see Chapter 31). A dose of 5 mg per day has been suggested for osteoporosis prevention (as opposed to treatment), but the indications for this use of the drug are not well defined. Most physicians managing a patient who does not yet have clear indications for active drug treatment would recommend lifestyle changes, with a repeat DXA in two or more years to assess progress.

Alendronate (Fosamax) is now available in a combined pill for once weekly dosing containing 70 mg alendronate (Fosamax) and 2,800 units of vitamin D3 ("Fosavance"). A weekly alendronate (Fosamax) pill with a higher dose of vitamin D (5,600 units) is also available in some countries.

Risedronate (Actonel)

Risedronate (Actonel) differs from alendronate (Fosamax) only in the nitrogen-containing group at position R2 in the bisphosphonate molecule (see Figure 14). In initial studies in postmenopausal women, using a dose of 5 mg per day, bone mineral density increased 4–5% at the spine and 2–4% at the hip over three years compared with placebo (see Figure 15). Like alendronate (Fosamax), risedronate (Actonel) reduced vertebral fractures by about 50%, and hip fractures to a similar extent in women with severe osteoporosis. A dose of 35 mg once weekly was approved in 2003, and appears to be similar to weekly alendronate (Fosamax).

It is approved for postmenopausal and glucocorticoid-induced osteoporosis.

Risedronate (Actonel) appears not to be very different from alendronate (Fosamax) in terms of side-effects, though gastro-intestinal side-effects such as heartburn and pain on swallowing may be modestly less with risedronate (Actonel). Risedronate (Actonel) 75 mg taken on two consecutive days per month has recently been shown to be as effective, at least with respect to changes in the bone mineral density, as 5 mg taken daily, and this preparation was approved by Health Canada in 2007.

Surprisingly, patient adherence to both alendronate (Fosamax) and risedronate (Actonel) is not particularly good. In the original studies, side-effects were few and inability to tolerate the drug was similar to placebo. However, abdominal pain and various dyspeptic symptoms are frequently attributed by patients to bisphosphonates. These or other symptoms, or other reasons, lead to discontinuation of the bisphosphonate in about 50% of patients within one year, most often in the first three months. Not surprisingly, it has been shown that patients who do not take the prescribed doses of the drugs do not get the full benefit. It is anticipated that bisphosphonates that can be taken less frequently, and probably those which can be administered by occasional injection, may be associated with better patient adherence than the earlier bisphosphonates.

Ibandronate (Boniva)

Ibandronate (Boniva) is another bisphosphonate which has been shown to increase bone mineral density to a similar extent as risedronate (Actonel) when given as a daily dose of 2.5 mg. A 50% reduction in new vertebral fractures was observed in patients with baseline compression fractures. One hundred and fifty mg by mouth once monthly appears to be as effective as 2.5 mg daily, based on measurements of bone markers, and has been approved in the US.

Zoledronic acid (Aclasta)

Zoledronic acid (Aclasta) is the most potent bisphosphonate currently available for clinical use, and has been used intravenously for certain complications of cancer and some rare bone diseases. Its potency stems from the combination of a very high tendency to bind to bone mineral, plus very high potency in suppressing osteoclasts. A single 4 or 5 mg intravenous dose reduces bone turnover for one year, so trials have been undertaken of its use in this manner (an annual intravenous infusion) for the treatment of osteoporosis.

The first large trial of zoledronic acid (Aclasta) in postmenopausal osteoporosis used a once yearly 5 mg dose, and demonstrated improvement in bone mineral density and a reduction in fractures, which has now been followed for up to three years (see Figure 15). At three years there was a 70% reduction in vertebral fractures and a 41% reduction in hip fractures. In a more recent trial, a 5 mg zoledronic acid (Aclasta) intravenous infusion was given to men and women with an average age of 76 years, within 90 days of surgery for a hip fracture. Compared with the placebo group, the zoledronic acid treated patients showed a significant reduction in subsequent fractures, by 30–50% at two years. Remarkably, there were also significantly fewer deaths in the zoledronic acid treated group, suggesting a mortality benefit for this agent in this particular patient group. It has recently been shown that the reduction in mortality cannot be entirely explained by the reduction in fractures, so zoledronic acid may have some other unrelated beneficial effects. These may prove to be very important results.

Intravenous bisphosphonates can cause kidney damage if given too rapidly, so zoledronic acid is generally given over 15 minutes rather than all at once. Between 10 and 30% of patients suffer from fever and muscle pain (flu-like symptoms) after the first injection, which may be decreased by pre-treatment with an anti-inflammatory or glucocorticoid, but the symptoms rarely occur with subsequent injections.

A single 5 mg intravenous dose of zoledronic acid (Aclasta) costs approximately $700 CDN. This is in comparison with an annual cost for weekly alendronate (Fosamax) or risedronate (by mouth) of about $300, but it is less than 10% of the cost of one year of teriparatide (Forteo). Patient adherence, by virtue of the route of administration, will, of course, be much better than has been seen with oral bisphosphonates.

Long-term use and safety of bisphosphonates

As noted above, ongoing regular administration of alendronate (Fosamax) continues to increase bone mineral density for at least ten years. In terms of potency in improving bone mineral density, it is more effective than calcitonin or raloxifene (Evista) (see below), but less so than teriparatide (Forteo) or parathyroid hormone. There are no direct comparisons of efficacy for fracture prevention.

There have been theoretical concerns that prolonged suppression of bone turnover, and increased bone mineralization might lead to stiffer and more brittle bone—so-called "frozen bone", and some have suggested periodic withdrawal of bisphosphonates or "drug holidays". However, bisphosphonates are firmly bound in the bones, and it may take at least five years for bone turnover to fully recover from a course of some bisphosphonates. At this time, there is little or no evidence to support these concerns. Bone turnover is not abolished with usual doses of bisphosphonates; an additional dose of a potent bisphosphonate in a treated patient causes further suppression of bone turnover markers, indicating a persisting low background level of bone turnover, which is presumably sufficient to maintain bone health. Although the frequency of fractures has not been found to rise after long-term bisphosphonate treatment (so there is no evidence to suggest the development of brittle bone) there have been a few cases reported of patients on bisphosphonates having fractures in unusual sites (less common types of hip fractures), suggesting that it may be prudent not to continue these drugs longer than is necessary (see below).

The issue of osteonecrosis of the jaw has already been discussed; it is being closely monitored but the very small risk is not felt at present to outweigh the obvious benefits of bisphosphonates in osteoporosis. The incidence with oral alendronate (Fosamax) is less than one case per 100,000 years of treatment (eg. one case would develop in a total of ten thousand patients each treated for 10 years). Two possible cases were reported in the initial large zoledronic acid study involving about four thousand patients—one in a zoledronic acid treated patient and one in the placebo group! It is presently recommended that patients receiving bisphosphonates have their usual regular dental visits. No special examination is required before starting treatment, and dental implants are not contra-indicated. There is no evidence to support stopping the bisphosphonate before dental procedures, although this has been recommended in some guidelines developed by the dental profession.

The use of bisphosphonates in combination with other drugs in osteoporosis has not been thoroughly studied. It was predicted that parathyroid hormone (PTH) or teriparatide (Forteo) and bisphosphonate in combination might be more potent than either alone. However, in early studies, teriparatide (Forteo) was less effective when given to the patient already receiving a bisphosphonate than to the "treatment naïve" patient. However, unless a course of PTH or teriparatide (Forteo) is followed by a course of an antiresorptive drug such as a bisphosphonate, the gains in bone mineral density from the PTH or teriparatide (Forteo) are rapidly lost.

Further studies are needed to determine the optimal duration of bisphosphonate treatment. In one of the few studies examining this issue, in postmenopausal women with osteoporosis who had been treated for five years with alendronate (Fosamax), 10 mg daily, the alendronate (Fosamax) was either discontinued, or continued at a dose of 5 or 10 mg daily for a further five years. The bone mineral density fell slowly in those in whom alendronate (Fosamax) was discontinued, and bone markers increased, indicating an increase in bone turnover. There was no difference in non-vertebral fractures, or in X-ray detected vertebral fractures, but there were more clinically recognized painful fractures in the women who discontinued the alendronate (Fosamax). One of the reasons why the differences were so small is probably the fact that bisphosphonates are strongly bound to bone, and after administration of the drug is stopped, it is slowly released from the remodeling bone and reattaches to the bone mineral so that its effect may continue long-term. It was concluded that discontinuation does not increase fracture risk in most patients, and so discontinuation may be appropriate in patients who are not actively fracturing. Those with continuing vertebral fractures or very low bone mineral densities may benefit from continuation, or perhaps from switching to an alternative drug.

In patients remaining on bisphosphonates, there is not yet evidence to show if continuation beyond 10 years confers additional benefit. It should also be kept in mind that the long-term effects of other bisphosphonates, or those given intravenously, could differ from those of oral alendronate (Fosamax).

Bisphosphonates, therefore, are very effective in osteoporosis, and are likely to remain a keystone of treatment for a long time to come. More research is needed to define the optimal duration of treatment and the indications for changing to one of the available alternative treatments. It is quite possible that intermittent bisphosphonate treatment will prove to be as effective as continuous treatment in appropriate patients, particularly in view of the continuing effect after administration ceases. These complex issues have not yet been addressed in good clinical studies; consequently opinions are based on the current understanding of bone biology and how bisphosphonates have acted so far.

Other uses of bisphosphonates

Bisphosphonates are used for bone scanning, by attaching a radioactive label (technetium) to the bisphosphonate. The labeled bisphosphonate is given by intravenous injection, and is taken up preferentially by areas of bone where turnover is increased, such as some secondary cancers and healing recent fractures. A scanning machine is then used to find the "hot spots" where the bisphosphonate has accumulated.

Bisphosphonates are used in the treatment of Paget's disease of the bone, a disorder in which osteoclasts multiply excessively and are abnormally active, leading to local and sometimes painful bone lesions. Bisphosphonates are the preferred treatment for most clinical problems related to Paget's disease of the bone.

Bisphosphonates are used to treat various complications of cancer, including bone invasion by the cancer, and hypercalcemia (high blood calcium) secondary to cancer, and they have become the treatment of choice (often given intravenously) in these situations, in which they may prolong life. It is in these intravenous bisphosphonate-treated cancer patients that osteonecrosis of the jaw, which has recently come under scrutiny as a possible complication of bisphosphonate treatment in osteoporosis, has mainly occurred.

CHAPTER TWENTY

Parathyroid hormone and teriparatide (Forteo)

A PROTEIN IS A CHAIN OF BUILDING BLOCKS called amino acids arranged in a particular unique sequence. The parathyroid glands and the hormone they secrete—parathyroid hormone (PTH) were discussed in detail in Chapter 13 in the section "Understanding calcium metabolism". PTH is a protein consisting of a chain of 84 amino-acids; teriparatide (Forteo) is the name given to the man-made amino acid chain which comprises the first 34 amino acids (1–34) of PTH. This fragment has all of the biological activity of the whole (1–84) PTH molecule, including the anabolic effect on bone (see below).

Parathyroid hormone and teriparatide (Forteo) represent a novel approach to the treatment of osteoporosis since, unlike bisphosphonates and other available treatments, they are not antiresorptive but instead increase new bone formation (known as an anabolic effect) and also they can improve trabecular microarchitecture. The bone building effect of daily teriparatide (Forteo) injections was first demonstrated in humans in 1980, although this property of PTH had been demonstrated in experimental animals in the 1930s.

Most clinical studies have used teriparatide (Forteo); although it is anticipated that the anabolic effects of PTH and teriparatide (Forteo) will be the same. Teriparatide (Forteo) increases the remodeling rate and increases the amount of bone deposited in each bone remodeling unit. This can increase trabecular thickness. Bone formation can occur without resorption, perhaps by activating quiescent lining cells to form active osteoblasts. Trabecular connectivity has been shown to improve with teriparatide (Forteo) treatment.

Treatment with teriparatide (Forteo) increases both bone formation and resorption within a few weeks, as reflected by changes in bone markers, the increase in formation occurring first. As discussed earlier, the bone building effect of teriparatide (Forteo), whereby bone mineral density is increased, may involve the stimulation of osteoblastic activity.

The original studies of teriparatide (Forteo) in postmenopausal women with vertebral fractures showed that 18 months of daily subcutaneous injections in doses of 20 or 40 micrograms per day resulted in an increase in bone mineral density of 9.7% and 13.7% respectively at the spine, with lesser increases at the hip. Vertebral fractures were reduced by 65% and 69%, and non vertebral fragility fractures by 50%. The risk of moderate or severe compression fractures was reduced by 90%. The fracture risk reduction was independent of age, initial bone mineral density or the presence of pre-existing vertebral fractures. This study was stopped because experiments in rats had shown that very large doses of teriparatide (Forteo) could cause a form of bone cancer (osteosarcoma). Subsequently this was shown not to occur in rats given lower doses, more comparable with those used in humans, or in other animal species. Moreover, this type of bone cancer has been reported only once in 250,000 treated patients.

The main side-effects of teriparatide (Forteo) were leg cramps, dizziness and irritation at the injection sites. A small increase in the serum calcium level is often seen, peaking at 4–6 hours after the injection, but very rarely sufficient to cause concern. If it is felt to be excessive, either the teriparatide (Forteo) dose can be reduced, or calcium supplements decreased. Twenty-four hour urinary calcium may also increase, and this may be a concern in patients with a history of calcium-containing kidney stones.

It has been suggested that severe vitamin D deficiency should be excluded, at least in patients in whom there is good reason to suspect it, by measuring the 25(OH)D level before starting teriparatide (Forteo) treatment. An increase in uric acid concentration occurs in a few patients, and gout has been reported.

Increases in bone mineral density with teriparatide (Forteo) were greatest in trabecular bone, and least in cortical bone, averaging 10–14% over three years at the spine (see Figure 15), and 5% over three years at the femoral neck. In direct comparisons with alendronate (Fosamax), markers of bone formation increased with teriparatide (Forteo) but decreased with alendronate (Fosamax). Increases in bone mineral density were greater with teriparatide (Forteo) than alendronate (Fosamax), particularly in the spine.

In men with osteoporosis, in glucocorticoid-induced osteoporosis, and in acute estrogen deficiency due to nafarelin treatment (a drug used to reduce estrogen levels in women), teriparatide (Forteo) improves bone mineral density in the spine and femoral neck.

All of the above studies have employed teriparatide (Forteo). Limited studies with intact PTH suggest that it has similar efficacy to teriparatide (Forteo). PTH is not yet available for the treatment of osteoporosis in Canada, but has been used in some clinical studies in the US. Both agents have been given by daily subcutaneous injection. Benefiting from the technology developed for insulin injection in diabetics, it is extremely easy for patients to learn to administer their own daily injection.

Teriparatide (Forteo) in combination with bisphosphonate

Because many patients with severe fracturing osteoporosis, and in need of effective additional treatment, are already receiving a bisphosphonate, many studies have been done exploring this combination to see if the effects are additive. Although results are complicated, a reasonable summary would be that prior bisphosphonate blunts, but does not abolish, the beneficial effect of teriparatide (Forteo) or PTH.

When teriparatide (Forteo) that has been given alone for 12–18 months is stopped, the gains in bone mineral density are rapidly lost unless preventative treatment is given. Studies have shown that a course of alendronate (Fosamax) for one year, after one year of teriparatide (Forteo) or PTH, not only prevents losses but adds to the gains. It is therefore now recommended that a course of teriparatide (Forteo) or PTH be followed by a bisphosphonate such as alendronate (Fosamax) or risedronate (Actonel) in the usual doses for at least one year, and probably much longer. Studies are under way to define effective regimens, which might involve intermittent rather than continuous bisphosphonate treatment after the course of teriparatide (Forteo).

Who should get teriparatide (Forteo)?

At a cost of approximately $10,000 per year, teriparatide (Forteo) is significantly more expensive than bisphosphonates and other antiresorptive treatments for osteoporosis.

Potential candidates for PTH therapy include:

1. Patients who are fracturing despite bone mineral density levels above the traditional cut-off for diagnosing osteoporosis (T-score greater than −2.5). This is because the effectiveness of teriparatide (Forteo) appears to be unrelated to the number of pre-existing fractures and to the reduction in bone mineral density before therapy. Bisphosphonates on the other hand, are more effective in patients with more severe osteoporosis which is indicated by pre-existing fractures and severe reductions in bone mineral density.

2. Patients with very low bone mineral density. Because of its rapid effect, teriparatide (Forteo) may be particularly appropriate in patients with a very high fracture risk, associated with a T-score of less than −3.5. However, there has been no clinical trial yet that proves that teriparatide (Forteo) is more effective than bisphosphonates in preventing fractures in these circumstances.

3. Unsatisfactory response to bisphosphonates. This would particularly include patients with low bone mineral density, who do not respond to bisphosphonates and who experience continuing fracturing. In such patients, secondary causes of osteoporosis such as vitamin D deficiency and other endocrine disorders need to be ruled out. At present there is no evidence from clinical trials that these patients will necessarily respond better to teriparatide (Forteo), but uncontrolled observations in small numbers of patients suggest that this may be the case. Intolerance to bisphosphonates (usually due to gastro-intestinal side-effects) might now lead to a trial of intravenous bisphosphonate rather than the more expensive option of teriparatide (Forteo).

4. Because the evidence for prevention of vertebral fractures by teriparatide (Forteo) is stronger than hip and other non-vertebral fractures, in some jurisdictions it is mainly used for people with vertebral fractures.

Teriparatide (Forteo) has been shown to be effective in post-menopausal women and in men over 50. It is probably not appropriate for younger individuals with low bone mineral density, since their fracture risk is much lower than in older persons. Safety in pregnancy has not been demonstrated. Teriparatide is not recommended in adolescents and patients previously treated with radiotherapy, because of an increased risk for the development of osteosarcoma (bone cancer).

Teriparatide (Forteo) is approved for an 18 month course of treatment in Canada (two years in some other jurisdictions). Some physicians monitor the serum calcium after onemonth to exclude hypercalcemia.

Some alternatives to subcutaneous teriparatide (Forteo) or parathyroid hormone (PTH) are currently under investigation. There are also novel chemical forms of PTH. It is possible that teriparatide (Forteo) or PTH could be delivered transdermally (through the skin) or transnasally by nasal spray, and finally, it might be possible to provoke the patient's own parathyroid glands to produce a daily burst of PTH with the use of a new group of drugs (calcilytics) that interact with the calcium receptor on the parathyroid gland cells (see Chapter 12).

CHAPTER TWENTY-ONE

Raloxifene (Evista) and calcitonin

Raloxifene (Evista)

RALOXIFENE (EVISTA) BELONGS TO A GROUP OF DRUGS known as Selective Estrogen Receptor Modulators or "SERMs".

SERMs are medications that interact with estrogen (E2) receptors, causing stimulation or blocking in different tissues in which these receptors are found. A particular SERM may block receptors in one organ but stimulate receptors in another. Raloxifene (Evista) blocks the receptor E2 action in the breast and uterus (and therefore is not associated with increased risk of cancer of the breast or uterus) but stimulates estrogen's positive effect on bone.

Raloxifene (Evista) has been the subject of some very large studies. It increases spinal bone mineral density slightly, and reduces the risk for vertebral fracture by 40%, but has no effect on the risk of non-vertebral fractures. It is given as a single daily dose (60 mg) in pill form. There is some evidence to suggest that it may increase in the number of fatal strokes in patients compared with placebo controls. In addition, raloxifene (Evista) shares with estrogen a tendency to increase the risk of blood clots, including those in the legs and in the lungs, so anyone with a history of such events should not take raloxifene (Evista). Raloxifene (Evista) provides protection against breast cancer, reducing the risk by about 50% and it has been approved for use in breast cancer prevention in some countries.

It is obviously very difficult to balance the potential benefits of raloxifene (Evista) with its risks when treating osteoporosis. Because there are now several alternative treatments available, raloxifene (Evista) is being used less frequently. A remaining indication for its use is the patient's inability to tolerate other more potent treatments such as bisphosphonates.

Other SERMs are currently under investigation. One of these, Lasifoxifene, in large studies in post-menopausal women, has been shown to cause significant increases in bone density and reductions in vertebral and non-vertebral fractures. So far it has not been associated with increases in stroke or coronary heart disease, and breast cancer was significantly reduced. As with raloxifene (Evista) and estrogen, it is associated with an increase in blood clots.

Calcitonin

Calcitonin, like PTH, is a natural protein hormone involved in the control of calcium metabolism (see Chapter 14). It was initially hoped that it would prove to be a useful treatment for osteoporosis as well as other bone diseases. It was first given by injection, but because it is absorbed across mucus membranes, it is now often given by nasal spray. There have been several studies of the usefulness of calcitonin in osteoporosis. In late postmenopausal women (more than five years after menopause) nasal spray calcitonin was found to increase spinal bone mineral density by 1–2% over two years. There is evidence that vertebral fractures are significantly reduced. Uniquely among osteoporosis treatments, calcitonin provides significant pain relief in vertebral fractures.

If calcitonin has a role in the treatment of osteoporosis, it is probably in late postmenopausal women, especially where acute vertebral fracture pain is a major problem, and where other treatments cannot be tolerated. It remains in use for the treatment of acute pain in osteoporosis, but it has been largely replaced by the more potent and convenient bisphosphonates. For osteoporosis, it is given as 200 units daily in alternate nostrils, or 100 units per day by injection. Side-effects are mild and include nasal irritation (rhinitis) and, when given by injection, flushing of the face. If significant benefit is not seen within two weeks calcitonin should be replaced by other treatments.

CHAPTER TWENTY-TWO

Strontium ranelate and other medications

Strontium ranelate

STRONTIUM IS A CHEMICAL ELEMENT closely related to calcium, which can replace calcium in the bone mineral. Strontium is best known because of its isotope Strontium 90 which is one of the radioactive products of nuclear fission (of uranium atoms). The non-radioactive isotope that occurs most commonly in nature and is present in strontium ranelate, is Strontium 88.

Strontium ranelate is a strontium compound which is given by mouth in a dose of 2 grams per day. Strontium is taken up by bone, particularly newly formed bone. After stopping treatment, the strontium is fairly rapidly released from the bone (unlike bisphosphonates). In postmenopausal women with osteoporosis and at least one vertebral compression fracture, when compared with placebo it decreased bone resorption and perhaps also increased bone formation, resulting in an increase in bone mineral density and an approximately 50% reduction in the risk of vertebral fractures, beginning in year 1, and continuing through year five of the treatment. Vertebral fractures were assessed by careful comparison of annual spine X-rays, and showed a 24% reduction in patients taking strontium ranelate compared with placebo, while the risk of hip fracture decreased by 43%.

Unlike the pure antiresorptive agents such as bisphosphonates, strontium ranelate may have both anabolic and antiresorptive effects.

115

Because strontium has a higher atomic weight than calcium, the replacement of some bone calcium by strontium, increases the bone mineral density as measured by DXA, even if the actual bone mineral content is unchanged. Nearly 50% of the increase in bone mineral density seen in patients taking strontium ranelate can be attributed to the physical presence of the strontium itself, the remainder representing a true increase in bone mineral density.

Bone markers are suggestive of increased bone formation as well as decreased resorption. Recently strontium ranelate has been shown to have positive effects in patients who have been on long-term bisphosphonates, suggesting that it could be useful in the treatment of such patients.

Strontium ranelate is associated with very few side-effects. Diarrhea has been noted. There was some initial concern about blood clots as a possible side-effect, but this has not been confirmed. Recently a few cases have been reported of severe skin reactions (rashes) in patients taking strontium ranelate; it is recommended that the drug be stopped immediately if a rash occurs.

Strontium ranelate is therefore a promising treatment with proven effectiveness as an inhibitor of bone resorption which may also promote bone formation. To date it has mainly been used in Europe. It is not yet released in Canada, but it is anticipated that it may become available in 2009. It is taken as one 2 gram sachet once daily, between meals. Other strontium-containing preparations such as strontium citrate can be obtained from some health food stores in Canada. However, their strontium content has been found to vary considerably, and their use is not recommended.

Fluoride

Fluoride has been known to have a powerful anabolic effect in bone for many decades, stimulating bone formation and increasing bone mineral density. In some areas, well water is heavily contaminated with fluoride, which leads to a generalized increase in bone mineral density of those consuming the water, sometimes affecting domestic animals such as dogs as well as humans. Fluoride can cause the formation of abnormal bone, including osteomalacia.

Fluoride is incorporated into the apatite crystals of bone, and may influence bone strength. In the doses in which it was used, there is no doubt that it increases bone mineral density, but results regarding fracture prevention are controversial. Smaller doses of fluoride, perhaps in combination with other agents, may provide greater fracture prevention, and are the subject of on-going research. However, at the present time, fluoride does not have an established place in the treatment of osteoporosis.

Denosumab

Monoclonal antibodies are laboratory-made antibodies which bind to specific proteins. Denosumab is a human monoclonal antibody that binds to a protein (called RANKL) which is involved in the formation of osteoclasts (see Appendix I). The end result is a decrease in bone resorption by osteoclasts.

In human studies, Denosumab has been given by subcutaneous injection every three or six months. Measurements of bone markers show that it causes a brisk decline in bone resorption. A recent study compared the effects of different doses given at different intervals with that of weekly alendronate (Fosamax). The dose of 30 mg every three months or 60 mg every six months appeared to be the most effective, and, in both cases the effect on bone mineral density was at least as great as that of alendronate (Fosamax). Unlike alendronate (Fosamax), Denosumab increased bone mineral density at the lower radius (forearm), which is mainly cortical bone, raising the hope that this new treatment might have greater anti-fracture effectiveness than other antiresorptive treatments for fractures involving a significant proportion of cortical bone, perhaps including hip fractures. The three-year results of a very large multi-national study of Denosumab in women aged 60–90 with an average T-score at the spine of –2.8 have shown a significant reduction in vertebral, non-vertebral and hip fractures in treated patients. Side-effects were mild. 6-monthly Denosumab appears to be a very promising new treatment for osteoporosis.

Beyond initial treatment

CHAPTER TWENTY-THREE

Patients who do not do well

WITH THE IMPRESSIVE ARRAY of effective treatments now available for osteoporosis, it might be expected that fractures could now be prevented in most patients. Unfortunately none of the available drugs completely prevent fractures, even under clinical trial conditions when patients are being closely monitored and are taking their medications properly. A significant proportion of patients with existing fractures do sustain new fractures while on osteoporosis treatment. Furthermore, drug discontinuation is unacceptably high, often due to adverse side-effects.

There is a lack of consensus on what constitutes a failure of osteoporosis therapy. A UK definition of an unsatisfactory response is "another fragility fracture despite adhering fully to treatment for one year, together with a decline in bone mineral density below the pre-treatment baseline".

A problem with definitions based only on bone mineral density is the weak correlation between changes in bone mineral density and fracture rate. In the early risedronate (Actonel) studies, vertebral fractures were more common in patients whose spinal bone mineral density decreased than in those in whom it increased. However, a greater magnitude of increase in bone mineral density was not associated with fewer fractures. Similarly neither changes in vertebral nor in hip bone mineral density predicted non-vertebral fracture.

Thus, only a small portion of the fracture prevention can be attributed to improved bone mineral density; 16% with alendronate (Fosamax), and even less for risedronate (Actonel) and raloxifene (Evista). The rest of the fracture prevention is not reflected in changes in bone mineral density, and presumably relates to changes in microstructure, frequency of activation of bone remodeling units (BRUs), mechanical properties of bone, etc. Other studies suggest that 50% of fracture reduction may relate to decreased remodeling (as indicated by biochemical markers, see Chapter 9). For anabolic agents such as parathyroid hormone (PTH) and teriparatide (Forteo), a larger proportion of the fracture prevention is attributable to increases in bone mineral density. In the case of strontium ranelate, changes in hip bone mineral density may explain up to 74% of fracture prevention.

These observations are very important in the context of patient follow-up during and after drug treatment. Patients on treatment are frequently referred to specialist Osteoporosis Clinics because their repeat bone mineral density is not showing the expected increase (such as that reported in the published trials). However, it is not at all clear that a poor bone mineral density response necessarily predicts a poor outcome (repeat fractures), and much more research is needed to develop practice guidelines for dealing with such patients. Similarly, it is important to realize that a declining risk of fracture does not mean that fracture risk is eliminated.

Treatment failure, as defined above, is clearly an indication to review the diagnosis to exclude secondary causes and to ensure adherence with lifestyle aspects of treatment and proper use of osteoporosis medications. If no clear explanation of the failure is identified, a change in medications should be considered. This usually means a change from a bisphosphonate to PTH, but as other treatments become available (such as strontium ranelate and Denosumab), indications for their use will be developed.

For a variety of reasons, up to 50% of patients may have an inadequate clinical response to treatment. A recent European study identified approximately equal numbers of patients who had either experienced a fragility fracture after at least 12 months of treatment (Group 1), or discontinued treatment (Group 2). These patients had severe osteoporosis (average T-score at spine −3.5) and a high incidence of previous fractures (68%). Group 1 tended to be older, less active, and to have had more falls. Quality of life tended to be lower in Group 1 than Group 2. Discontinuation of drugs due to side-effects was frequent with bisphosphonates (usually due to gastro-intestinal problems), and raloxifene (Evista).

Other studies have shown that failure to adhere to osteoporosis treatment can be as high as 50%, and non-compliant patients have a significantly greater fracture risk. These studies suggest that it may be possible to identify, at the commencement of treatment, patients who are more likely to have a poor clinical outcome, which would allow more resources to be expended on following up this group, focusing on lifestyle issues related to both osteoporosis and falls, and changing treatment if required. The problem of patient adherence is being addressed by developing bisphosphonates that can be given less frequently and perhaps by injection rather than by mouth. Adherence with a once yearly infusion, e.g. of zoledronic acid (Aclasta), is likely to be far better than adherence with a weekly bisphosphonate tablet, which may cause gastrointestinal side-effects. Similarly, adherence with 6-monthly injections of Denosumab, if and when this drug is released, would be expected to be very good.

Monitoring of biochemical bone markers (see Chapter 9) can be helpful in patient management, though it is not required routinely. Decreases in markers of resorption precede decreases in formation markers when antiresorptive drugs such as bisphosphonates and SERMs are started, and the vertebral fracture reduction correlates with the short-term decrease in markers. The measurement of markers might also increase patient adherence, since the physician can show data to the patient which confirm that the treatment is having the desired effect, though this has not been proved to be the case in controlled studies.

CHAPTER TWENTY-FOUR

Management of fractures

Fracture healing in osteoporosis: Is it different?

THE HEALING OF FRACTURES is not adversely influenced in patients who also have osteoporosis. The orthopaedic management, generally involving some sort of immobilization to reduce pain and to allow the fracture to heal, is therefore not different in the osteoporotic from the non-osteoporotic fracture patient. There was earlier concern that bisphosphonates, widely used in the treatment of osteoporosis, might interfere with the healing of fractures, but the data from several large studies suggest that healing is normal.

Hip fractures

Fracture of the hip is the most serious consequence of osteoporosis and has a significant mortality; it is estimated that one quarter of women and one third of men die within one year of a hip fracture. There are many reasons for this, including reduced mobility leading to muscle atrophy, blood clots and pneumonia, and the requirement for surgery (and post-surgical complications). Many patients have residual pain or limited mobility even after surgical repair (fixation of the fracture). Early fixation of the fracture, within 48 hours, allows early weight-bearing and mobilization. Early mobilization is the key to decreasing complications and mortality. Those patients who do not have early surgery have a very high mortality rate following hip fracture.

Figure 16 shows an X-ray of a hip fracture through the neck of the femur (femoral neck), close to the hip joint. In this particular fracture, the bone on either side of the fracture has retained its position—that is there is no 'displacement' of the fracture. Often the bone on either side of the fracture will become more widely separated 'displaced' and such a fracture is more unstable.

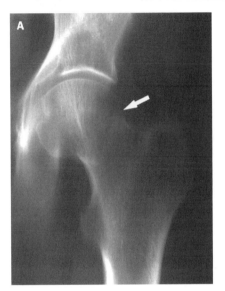 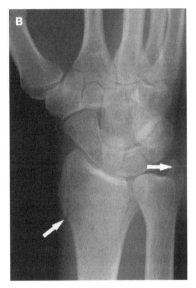

Figure 16: X-rays of hip and wrist fractures
(A) The hip, showing a fracture through the neck of the femur (femoral neck) without displacement. (B) The wrist, showing a fracture involving the lower ends of both forearm bones (radius and ulna).

The treatment of any fracture is to bring the broken ends of the bone together, in the right alignment, and then prevent the broken ends from moving relative to one another. If the ends of the fracture continually move, healing is delayed. The treatment step in which the ends are 'fixed' together to prevent them from moving is called 'fixation'. There are many different ways of creating fixation of fractures, depending upon what bone is broken. For example, a simple plaster cast may be all that is required for fixation of an arm or leg fracture. The anatomy of the hip, however, makes it a much more difficult fracture site for fixation, but it is important that it be done if the complications of immobility are to be avoided.

Fixation of hip fractures to allow early weight-bearing is generally done in one of two ways. Either the hip is 'pinned', or a part of it (the head) is replaced with an artificial device (prosthesis). In pinning, metal screws or a bolt are placed across the fracture site in order to hold the ends of the fractured bone fixed against one another in good alignment. Alternatively, if the fracture site is high up towards the femoral head (ball) of the hip joint so that the blood supply of the head is damaged and there is risk of death of the femoral head due to interruption of its blood supply, the femoral head is replaced with a metal ball that fits into the socket normally occupied by the femoral head. This differs from "total hip replacement," which is the standard procedure for advanced arthritis of the hip joint, in that, with total hip replacement, both the socket and the head are replaced. In fracture management, there is rarely a need to replace the socket.

Patients suffering from a fragility fracture such as a low trauma hip fracture should be investigated and treated for osteoporosis. Unfortunately that is often not the case, so that the opportunity is frequently missed to start the patient on treatment that could reduce the risk of future fractures. In this context, a recent study giving a once yearly infusion of zoledronic acid (Aclasta) starting within three months of surgical treatment of a hip fracture is of great interest, as it demonstrated a significant reduction in the subsequent fractures, with very minor side-effects, and a reduction in mortality compared with patients not receiving the bisphosphonate.

Vertebral fractures

As already noted, vertebral fractures often do not cause any associated symptoms. They most commonly occur in the midthoracic (T6-8) and thoracolumbar (T12-L1) regions, but can occur at any level (Figure 5). They may vary in severity, and can have several different configurations:

1. Predominantly in the anterior (front) part of the vertebral body, causing it to become wedge-shaped, and contributing to forward curvature (kyphosis) — i.e. the spine above the fracture is angulated forwards on the spine below;

2. Complete, affecting the whole vertebral body, with the greatest risk of spinal cord compression; or

3. Biconcave, preserving the anterior and posterior heights of the vertebra, with collapse of the central portion.

Some vertebral fractures are painful and may require temporary bed rest. The cumulative results of several compression fractures can be devastating, with significant kyphosis of the spine and loss of height leading to serious deformity with accompanying loss of self esteem. With repeated fractures, the movements of the chest wall during breathing can become compromised, leading to respiratory problems. With the loss in height of the lumbar spine, the ribs may rest uncomfortably on the pelvic bone, and the abdomen may protrude forward. Balance may also be impaired, leading to falls and further fractures.

In most patients with a vertebral compression fracture, pain relief medications and modification of posture and activity are sufficient treatment, and the pain subsides in a few days. However, in a few patients, severe pain persists. Such patients may be candidates for a short trial of calcitonin treatment (see Chapter 14). Alternatively, minimally invasive surgical treatment—either vertebroplasty or kyphoplasty, may be considered (see below).

Surgery for vertebral fractures

In vertebroplasty, a needle is introduced from behind into the vertebral body, and bone cement (methyl methacrylate) is injected under high pressure. In kyphoplasty, an inflatable balloon is passed via the same route into the vertebral body and inflated in an effort to partially re-expand the vertebra and reduce the angulation. The balloon is then removed and the space filled with cement under lower pressure. On average, 30–40% of the lost height is regained.

Severe pain is the indication for these procedures. Almost 80% of patients with pain treated with these surgical procedures are said to experience dramatic pain relief. A recent randomized trial of balloon kyphoplasty showed a significantly improved quality of life and reduced back pain and disability, without an increase in the risk of further vertebral fractures over the first year, in kyphoplasty patients. Complications are very infrequent. A controlled study of the cosmetic benefit of kyphoplasty or vertebroplasty has not been reported; at the present time pain rather than deformity is the usual indication for these procedures.

CHAPTER TWENTY-FIVE

Physical Therapy in Osteoporosis*

THE PHYSIOTHERAPIST IS A KEY MEMBER of the osteoporosis health care team, along with the nurse, physician, dietician and occupational therapist. The input of the physiotherapist is important at all stages of osteoporosis management, from prevention of the disease, to the avoidance of falls and fractures, and to rehabilitation following fractures. Physiotherapists employ a wide range of treatment methods, including strength exercises, posture re-education, flexibility exercises, ergonomic advice, balance exercises, and many more.

There are five principal means by which physical therapy can help patients who have osteoporosis or who are at risk of developing it:

Promotion of bone formation

Regular weight bearing exercise contributes to the achievement of an optimal peak bone mass early in life, and may help to reduce

---

*Based on discussions with Dr. Meena Sran. Dr. Sran works for the Osteoporosis Program, BC Women's Health Centre, and is a Canadian Institutes of Health Research and Michael Smith Foundation for Health Research Post-doctoral Fellow. The publication "The Role of the Physical Therapist in the Prevention and Management of Osteoporosis" in the "Journal of Women's Health Physical Therapy", 29;3 2005 by Meena and Karim M Khan MD PHD (Dept of Family Practice, Faculty of Medicine, UBC) served as a reference paper for this chapter.

bone loss in later years. It is therefore important regardless of age. Beneficial activities include walking, jogging, Tai-chi, stair-climbing, dancing or tennis. Progressive resistance training such as exercises that include gradually increasing weights properly lifted, pushed or pulled, improves muscle strength and may reduce bone loss. Such training can significantly improve one's ability to carry out activities of daily living. For example, strengthening of the quadriceps muscles (front of the thigh) improves the ability to rise unassisted from a chair.

For the patient with established osteoporosis, it is important to avoid exercise that might increase the risk of falls or fractures (ice-skating, roller-blading, diving, skiing, hiking in rough terrain), but it is also important not to unnecessarily restrict patients and make them feel like invalids.

Education of the patient, together with an individualized exercise program is required, and the physiotherapist is best equipped to provide this advice. Physiotherapists with a particular knowledge of osteoporosis-related issues are increasingly available both in hospitals and in the community.

Weight bearing to promote bone formation must be safe and take account of the patient's history. Walking is suitable for most patients. Jumping helps bone formation, but must be appropriate to the patient's individual circumstances. Regular weight bearing exercise must be continued, otherwise the benefits are lost.

Fall prevention

A history of a fall in the previous year is a very important predictor of future falls. Muscle strength and balance should be assessed. A reasonable test of function is the 'timed up-and-go' test, in which the patient stands up from a chair without pushing off with the arms, walks three meters, turns around and returns to the seated position. Taking more than 15 seconds to do this is associated with an increased risk of falls. It is important to observe the patient carefully during the test in order to identify risk factors for future falls such as undiagnosed leg weakness, balance issues or gait problems.

There is good evidence that physiotherapy, including an individualized exercise program combining strength and balance training, reduces the frequency of falls. Balance exercises may be the most effective component. Tai-chi is thought to be one of the best in this regard. Mobility aids such as canes and walkers improve stability in appropriate cases.

Ergonomic advice, education and environmental modification (removal of loose rugs, changing the configuration of the bathroom or adding handrails, for instance) may all be appropriate. The patient should be given specific advice regarding avoidance of falls in high risk areas such as the bathroom and kitchen, preferably based upon a home visit by an occupational therapist. Occupational therapists are experts in assessing the physical interaction between an individual and their living or working environment, and coming up with solutions to make that interaction safer and easier.

Fracture prevention

Vertebral fractures are sometimes attributed to lifting and bending activities. Educating the patient on correct and incorrect body mechanics, and providing them with appropriate diagrams, can be very helpful. Particularly in patients with a previous history of a fracture, training should be given on how to bend and lift properly (e.g. avoidance of lifting or exercising with the back bent), as well as avoidance of twisting the trunk. The physiotherapist can give specific advice on activities such as gardening, computer use, child care (particularly lifting children), and housework. Simple ergonomic aids such as kneeling pads for gardening and an ergonomic computer station may be appropriate. Hip protectors, as discussed earlier, may be useful in individuals with a high risk of falling.

Post-fracture rehabilitation

Fractures of the wrist or hip are generally obvious and require emergency orthopedic treatment, followed by graduated exercise and, where necessary, mobility aids, ergonomic advice and environmental modification to facilitate optimal rehabilitation. The period of immobilization should be kept to a minimum as it may lead to increasing muscle weakness and worsening of osteoporosis.

Vertebral compression fractures vary greatly with respect to accompanying symptoms. If pain is severe it will require pain-relieving medications. A number of other types of treatment may help the pain, including relaxation techniques, gentle massage, light muscle exercises, acupuncture, ultrasound, or a brace or corset. A brace, corset or other support device should only be used as a temporary measure as these may lead to further muscle weakness and increasing osteoporosis if worn too long. When pain is severe and persistent, vertebroplasty or kyphoplasty should be considered (see Chapter 24).

Treatment of other conditions that may be limiting mobility or may contribute to falls

Many patients with osteoporosis have other independent medical conditions that can predispose to osteoporosis or lead to falls that can result in a fracture. These may include underlying neurological problems such as a stroke (causing muscle weakness or impaired balance), side-effects of medications, visual impairment (bifocals and graduated lenses can cause problems seeing stairs adequately), consumption of alcohol, extreme cases of malnutrition or chronic depression with reduced mobility, etc. Often, multiple risk factors for falls are present. It is important that these conditions not be overlooked as, unrecognized, they can lead to failure of progress in managing osteoporosis.

Not just an older woman's problem

CHAPTER TWENTY-SIX

Osteoporosis in the premenopausal woman

MOST OF THE DISCUSSION IN EARLIER CHAPTERS focused on the post-menopausal woman, in whom osteoporosis is most common. However, low bone mass and fractures also occur in pre-menopausal women, in men, and rarely in children.

Much of what has been discussed earlier is applicable to pre-menopausal as well as postmenopausal women. This chapter will focus on those aspects of osteoporosis that require special attention when the patient is a premenopausal woman.

Does premenopausal osteoporosis require a different definition?

We have seen that postmenopausal osteoporosis has traditionally been defined on the basis of a T-score of –2.5 or less on bone mineral density testing, or a fragility fracture. The T-score relates the patient's bone mineral density to that of normal young adult women.

We have also seen that age is an important determinant of fracture risk. For a given bone mineral density, a premenopausal woman has a much lower 10-year fracture risk than an older woman, and it is agreed that osteoporosis should not be diagnosed in premenopausal women on the basis of the T-scores that are used in postmenopausal women. Rather, it is suggested that the Z-score (obtained by comparing the patient with values from age matched normal women) be used.

A Z-score lower than –2.0 should be described as "low bone mineral density", avoiding the use of the term osteoporosis in the premenopausal woman, except in the case of patients with a fragility fracture or secondary osteoporosis. The fracture risk associated with a Z-score of less than 2.0 is not clearly defined. The move away from the diagnostic use of T-scores and Z-scores and towards the use of a comprehensive fracture risk assessment tool (such as the FRAX® tool, discussed in detail in Chapter 11), may provide an alternative approach to this issue in the future. At present, however, the FRAX® tool is only applicable to postmenopausal women and men aged over 50.

Bone mineral density in premenopausal women

Bone mineral density is a result of the peak bone mass achieved, and any subsequent losses. Bone mass increases rapidly during the adolescent years, and is usually complete by age 20, within 4 years of the onset of menstruation. Earlier onset of menstrual periods is associated with a greater peak bone mass. Genetic factors, as well as nutrition, exercise, illness and medications are some factors that can limit peak bone mass. Factors which can increase premenopausal bone loss include ovulation disorders leading to a decrease in estrogen and progesterone, low body weight, insufficient calcium intake, alcohol consumption, smoking and a family history of osteoporosis.

The impact of pregnancies on bone mass is controversial, however, significant reversible bone loss accompanies lactation, presumably due to estrogen suppression and calcium losses in the milk.

Occasional patients present with fragility fractures and severe osteoporosis around the time of delivery or soon after. It is often unclear whether such patients have had osteoporosis for a long time and have had increased bone resorption associated with pregnancy which has further weakened the bone or whether they are otherwise normal women in whom pregnancy and/or lactation have caused much greater losses of bone mineral density than usual.

Premenopausal women who do suffer from fractures, including stress fractures, tend to have lower bone mineral densities, and women who suffer premenopausal fractures have a higher incidence of postmenopausal fractures.

It is important to note that a much higher proportion of premenopausal than postmenopausal women with a low bone mineral density have secondary osteoporosis, that is, there is an identifiable underlying cause, such as an underlying disease or medication. In the premenopausal patient, these possible causes should be carefully considered. Table 3 lists some of these causes of secondary osteoporosis; laboratory investigations are often required for their identification and treatment.

Table 3 **Causes of secondary osteoporosis in premenopausal women**
Hypogonadism (inadequate sex hormone levels)
Hyperparathyroidism
Hyperthyroidism
Vitamin D and/or calcium deficiency
Gastrointestinal malabsorption (e.g. celiac disease, postoperative states)
Anorexia nervosa,
Idiopathic (cause unknown) Hypercalciuria
Cushing's syndrome
Rheumatoid arthritis and other inflammatory conditions
Alcoholism
Renal (kidney) disease
Liver disease
Administration of excess thyroid hormone for treatment of hypothyroidism

Genetic diseases, including
    Osteogenesis imperfecta
    Marfan's syndrome
    Homocystinuria

Medications:
    Glucocorticoids (steroids)
    Immunosuppressants (e.g. cyclosporine)
    Antiseizure medications, particularly phenobarbital and phenytoin
    GnRH agonists (when used to suppress ovulation)
    Heparin

Cancer chemotherapy
Depot medroxyprogesterone acetate

Management of premenopausal osteoporosis

As with postmenopausal osteoporosis, dietary calcium and vitamin D intake should be optimized, to around 1000 mg calcium and 1,000 units of vitamin D per day. Excess alcohol and smoking should be avoided. Regular weight bearing exercise should be undertaken, a normal body weight maintained, and anorexia nervosa avoided or treated. These lifestyle modifications have been shown to result in some improvement in bone mineral density.

Specific approaches are required for the secondary forms of osteoporosis, and may include:

- Hormonal treatment for menstrual disorders.
- Surgery for primary hyperparathyroidism.
- Discontinuation of medications that suppress estrogen production, such as the treatment of endometriosis by nafarelin (Synarel).
- In young women with osteoporosis due to anorexia nervosa, generally associated with cessation of menstruation, bone loss can be very rapid and severe. The low bone density can persist into adult life. Combination estrogen-progesterone treatment is not effective in increasing bone mineral density. Instead, weight gain and resumption of normal menstrual function are necessary for recovery of bone mass. Oral bisphosphonates are under study but are not yet of proven benefit in increasing bone mineral density in patients with anorexia nervosa. IGF-1 (see Appendix II), an anabolic hormone which is produced in the liver and is deficient in anorexia nervosa is currently being explored as a possible treatment for osteoporosis associated with this condition.

Special considerations regarding drug treatment for the premenopausal osteoporosis patient

- SERMs such as raloxifene (Evista) are not used in premenopausal women because of concern about possible birth defects in the event of pregnancy.
- Calcitonin has not been shown to be effective in this group of patients.
- Bisphosphonates are a concern in reproductive age women, as these drugs can accumulate in fetal bones. They have been

used for glucocorticoid-induced osteoporosis (see Chapter 31), osteoporosis associated with anorexia nervosa, and for chemotherapy-associated osteoporosis, in which bone loss can be rapid if the treatment induces a premature menopause.

- Teriparatide (Forteo) has been shown to be effective in preventing bone loss in premenopausal women, but is not approved for that purpose in Canada.

Overall, the treatment options for the premenopausal woman are limited. Taken together with the usually fairly low absolute fracture risk, few premenopausal women are given active drug therapy for a low bone mineral density.

CHAPTER TWENTY-SEVEN

Osteoporosis in men

OSTEOPOROSIS IN MEN, though less common than in women, is a major problem which is seriously under-recognized and under-treated. Overall, osteoporotic fractures are about one half as common in men as in women. About one third of all hip fractures occur in men, with a mortality rate of nearly 40%, greater than that of women. About 20% of men who suffer a hip fracture subsequently have a second hip fracture. In a recent Canadian study, vertebral deformities were equally common in men and in women over age 50, at about 22%.

Normal men reach their peak bone mass somewhat later than women, but achieve a slightly higher peak, with larger bones. Thereafter bone mass declines with age, without the accelerated decline after the menopause, but with accelerated loss after about age 70, particularly in the presence of hypogonadism, in which cortical bone is preferentially lost. Hypogonadism means reduced ('hypo' means 'low') production of sex hormones by the testicles (gonads). Hypogonadism is a common problem amongst older men. In men, the integrity of the trabeculae is better preserved than in women, though they become thinner with aging. Thus, on average, men reach old age with a greater bone mass, larger bones and more intact trabeculae than women, and these are probably important reasons for their lower fracture rates. Men also have a shorter life expectancy than women.

Men have more fractures than women during childhood and adolescence, including fractures of limbs and vertebrae, perhaps related to their exposure to more trauma. After age 70, there is a marked increase in vertebral and hip fractures, which on average occur 5–10 years later in men than in women. There are racial differences in fractures, for example black males have fewer fractures than white males.

Causes of secondary osteoporosis in men

There is a higher incidence of secondary osteoporosis in men than in postmenopausal women. It is estimated that up to 60% of men with osteoporosis have associated medical conditions contributing to their osteoporosis. In the remainder, including many younger men, the osteoporosis is "primary", and it is assumed that, as in women, heredity plays a major role in this group.

The most common causes of secondary osteoporosis in men are hypogonadism, alcohol abuse and glucocorticoid use. Both male and female sex hormones—testosterone and estrogen—are produced by men and both are important for the male skeleton. Lack of male gonadal function can occur in old age and contribute to osteoporosis. Studies of elderly male residents of nursing homes have found that up to 66% of those with hip fractures and 20% of those with vertebral fractures have hypogonadism. Lack of testosterone can also result from certain drug treatments that are designed to reduce testosterone levels. Most commonly these are the anti-androgen treatments for prostate cancer (LHRH analogs). These agents are widely used because prostate cancer is relatively common, and the indications for using LHRH analogs are becoming broader. Such treatment may result in a rapid loss of bone mineral density unless steps are take to prevent it.

Normal men convert some testosterone (male hormone) into estrogen (female hormone). Research has shown that bone mineral density in men relates much more closely to estrogen level than testosterone level. Estrogen is known to be important in suppressing bone resorption by osteoclasts. Men who have an impairment in converting testosterone into estrogen develop osteoporosis, which responds to estrogen treatment. There appears to be a minimum threshold level of estrogen required for bone health (to suppress resorption of bone) in both men and women. With aging, members of both sexes may fall below that threshold level and begin losing bone.

Vitamin D deficiency may also contribute to osteoporosis. It was recently shown that the risk of hip fracture is higher in both men and women with 25(OH)D levels less than 62.5 nmol/L (25 ng/ml).

Evaluation of osteoporosis in men

The presence of a fragility fracture, or any condition known to predispose to osteoporosis, has generally been regarded as an indication for a bone mineral density measurement in a man. Some jurisdictions have recommended bone mineral density measurements in all men at 65 or 70 years of age or older.

Fewer men that women receive bone mineral density assessment following a fragility fracture, and so miss the opportunity to begin treatment for osteoporosis. Reasons for this relative neglect of male osteoporosis include lack of awareness among the public and medical profession that osteoporosis is common in men, and perhaps the stigma associated in mens' minds with having a 'woman's disease'.

Until recently, T-scores derived from bone densitometry at the hip in older men were interpreted as in postmenopausal women. T-scores were compared with young normal male values. A score of less than –2.5 was diagnosed as osteoporosis, and a score of –1.0 to –2.5 as osteopenia. Using these definitions for osteoporosis and osteopenia, the respective prevalences in older men are about 6% and 47%, and in women about 18% and 50%, confirming that osteoporosis is more common in women. The limitations of the diagnosis of osteopenia have been discussed previously, and Osteoporosis Canada now recommends that a T-score of –1.0 to –2.5 in a man over 50 years old be described simply as "reduced bone mineral density" rather than being given a diagnosis.

Osteoporosis Canada recommends that, in men less than 50 years old, as in younger women, Z-scores be used rather than T-scores, and that a Z-score greater than –2.0 be described as "within the expected range for age" while a score of less than –2.0 be described as "below the expected range for age".

As in the case of women, the majority of fractures occur in men whose bone mineral density is not in the osteoporotic range. Although bone mineral density is a strong indicator of fracture risk, prediction of fracture risk can be greatly improved by taking other factors into account, including:

- Age;
- Low BMI (body mass index);
- Prior fragility fracture at over age 50;
- Parental history of hip fracture;
- Current smoking;
- Use of systemic glucocorticoids for more than three months;
- Excessive alcohol use (three or more drinks per day);
- Rheumatoid arthritis.

The new FRAX® tool, discussed in Chapter 11 and currently applicable to postmenopausal women and men over 50 years of age assigns weight to each of these risk factors, and determines the 10-year fracture risk, with or without a bone mineral density measurement at the femoral neck.

As for women, it is anticipated that the FRAX® tool will be used in the future to help to determine who should have a bone mineral density measurement, and the 10-year fracture index (based on the above risk factors), with or without the femoral neck bone mineral density measurement, will be used to guide clinical decision–making, particularly drug treatment. In men, additional risk factors that could be included in the FRAX® tool in the future, if they were shown to independently predict fracture, include testosterone, estrogen and vitamin D levels.

Assessment of a male patient in whom osteoporosis is under consideration should include a clinical history and physical examination. Attention should be given to measurement of standing height as a baseline. A history of loss of height, increased spinal curvature (kyphosis), or a previous fragility fracture suggests significant osteoporosis. Evaluation also requires a review of dietary calcium and vitamin D intake, alcohol and smoking habits, medications that may increase the risk of falling such as sedatives and anticonvulsants, and level of physical activity including factors that may increase the risk of falls. It is important to assess what medications are being taken in order to identify those that can influence bone mass such as glucocorticoids and anticonvulsants or those might increase fracture risk such as certain antidiabetes medications (e.g. rosiglitazone) or proton pump inhibitors for stomach acid reflux. Finally, the family history for osteoporosis and fractures should be reviewed.

In the male patient with established osteoporosis on the basis of bone mineral density, appropriate additional laboratory testing is required to rule out secondary causes. Such tests may include measurement of blood calcium and PTH levels, tests of kidney and liver function, and tests to exclude thyroid disease, multiple myeloma, hypogonadism (testosterone or estrogen deficiency) and vitamin D deficiency. As in women, biochemical bone markers have not proved to be particularly useful for clinical management.

Vertebral fragility fractures are the most common fragility fracture, and a very strong risk factor for further fractures. The best method for identifying these fractures is a plain spinal X-ray, but in the patient having a bone mineral density, vertebral fracture assessment (VFA) will usually be included if the equipment software is available. This provides a reasonable view of the spine (not as good as a plain spinal X-ray but with less radiation).

Prevention of osteoporosis and fractures in men

Lifestyle issues, including recommended intakes of calcium (a total calcium intake of 1000–1500 mg per day is commonly recommended in men) and vitamin D (1000 units per day) are similar to women. Although controversial, a recent review suggested that 1200 mg calcium plus at least 800 units of vitamin D reduced fractures by 12% in both men and women over age 50. It is suggested that 25(OH)D levels should be 75 nmol/L (30 ng/ml) or higher. Appropriate steps should be taken to improve muscle strength, coordination and balance, in order to reduce the risk of falls.

Causes of secondary osteoporosis in men should be sought and treated

Testosterone replacement in hypogonadal men has been shown to increase spinal bone mineral density and improve the trabecular architecture of the bone (on MRI), but has not been shown to reduce fractures. The use of testosterone in men who are not hypogonadal is controversial, and it is not generally recommended. An increase in bone density has been reported with testosterone treatment. Muscle mass also increases, which may be very beneficial in elderly men with muscle wasting. Of concern with testosterone treatment are possible adverse effects on the cardiovascular system and the prostate gland. Analogous to SERMs, efforts are being made to develop SARMs—Selective Androgen Receptor Modulators— which it is hoped will retain the beneficial effects of testosterone (androgen) but not have the undesirable effects, and could be useful in the treatment of both male and female osteoporosis.

Since estrogens are very important for bone health in males, the possibility of preventing or treating osteoporosis with estrogens or related compounds is being studied. Long-term estrogen supplementation is not ideal because of the feminising effects of estrogen. However, SERMs (see Chapter 21) such as raloxifene (Evista) appear to have the positive bone effect of estrogen but not the feminising effect. Short-term studies of raloxifene in elderly men failed to show a significant reduction in bone resorption in the group as a whole, but there appeared to be a sub-group with low estrogen levels who did respond. Further studies are on-going to define the role for such treatment in male osteoporosis.

Bisphosphonates and teriparatide or PTH are effective in osteoporosis associated with hypogonadism, and may be more appropriate than testosterone for mild hypogonadism (in the absence of symptoms of testosterone lack) in elderly men.

As noted above, treatment of prostate cancer with LHRH analogs can cause rapid bone loss. These patients should usually have a baseline DXA determination of their bone density, which can be repeated periodically. Both oral and intravenous bisphosphonates have been used to try to preserve bone in these patients, and a large trial is currently underway using Denosumab.

Other secondary causes such as smoking and excessive alcohol intake are seen more often in men than in women and should be addressed.

The association of idiopathic hypercalciuria (increased calcium in the urine) with osteoporosis is better documented in men than women. Idiopathic hypercalciuria is usually discovered when a patient is found to have calcium-containing kidney stones, which leads to testing to determine if urinary calcium is elevated. This is not usually part of the routine investigation of male or female osteoporosis patients, but should be done in any osteoporosis patient with a history of kidney stones. There are some well studied patients of this type in whom bone mineral density improved significantly when the urinary calcium losses were controlled with a thiazide diuretic. Thus idiopathic hypercalciuria should be sought and treated in any patient presenting with the combination of kidney stones and a low bone mineral density.

Drug treatment of primary osteoporosis in men

The usual indication for drug treatment would be a fragility fracture, or a low bone mineral density. Traditionally, the threshold T-score of –2.5 has been used, but this should be replaced by a comprehensive fracture risk assessment using the FRAX® tool as soon as sufficient data are available.

Recent guidelines of the US National Osteoporosis Foundation recommend drug treatment in men 50 or older with a hip or vertebral fracture, men with a T-score below –2.5, and in men with a T-score between –1.0 and –2.5 with either a 10-year hip fracture probability of 3% or more, or a probability of any minimal trauma osteoporotic fracture of 20% or more (based on the locally adapted FRAX® algorithm). Earlier guidelines from Osteoporosis Canada were similar, and also included men with a T-score of –1.5 or less who are receiving glucocorticoid therapy for three months or more, or who have clinical hypogonadism. As with women, it is important to stress that these are only guidelines; each patient needs to be considered individually.

There have been far fewer studies of active drug treatments of osteoporosis in men than in women. However, alendronate (Fosamax) and risedronate (Actonel) increase bone mineral density in men (with or without hypogonadism) to a similar degree as in women, and there is evidence for a reduction in vertebral fractures. Alendronate (Fosamax), risedronate (Actonel) and etidronate (Didronel) have all been shown to be effective in glucocorticoid-induced bone loss in men. Following a hip fracture, a once yearly intravenous infusion of zoledronic acid (Aclasta) reduced clinical fractures and deaths in elderly men as well as women.

There have been no controlled trials with calcitonin in men.

Daily teriparatide (Forteo) injections are also highly effective in increasing bone mineral density in men with or without hypogonadism, and have been shown to reduce vertebral fractures. The improvement in BMD has been reported to be blunted by previous alendronate (Fosamax), but not risedronate (Actonel) treatment. In order to maintain the gain of bone mineral density, it is recommended that the usual 18 month course of teriparatide (Forteo) be followed by an oral bisphosphonate such as alendronate (Fosamax) or risedronate (Actonel).

There is a need for better data on the cost effectiveness of screening for and treatment of osteoporosis in men. A recent study addressing this issue suggested that a bone mineral density determination followed by five years of bisphosphonate therapy may be cost effective in US men with osteoporosis who are 65 or older and have had a previous clinical fracture, and for those 80 or older with no fracture. Additional studies are needed to determine how best to diagnose and treat men with osteoporosis within the general population.

PART THREE | **Being proactive**

SECTION NINE

Helping yourself

CHAPTER TWENTY-EIGHT

Do I have osteoporosis or am I developing it?

Why suspect osteoporosis?

MAINTAINING A 'HIGH LEVEL OF SUSPICION' about osteoporosis is important if an early diagnosis is to be made. It bears repeating that osteoporosis is a very common condition that causes no symptoms other than those associated with fractures, and even those may be painless. In the absence of a fragility fracture, it is possible to make a confident diagnosis of osteoporosis only by measuring the bone mineral density. Knowing what factors increase your risk for osteoporosis will alert you to the need to be proactive in seeking advice from your physician and possibly having a bone mineral density test or fracture risk assessment.

Risk factors for osteoporosis

A risk factor is something that increases your likelihood of having osteoporosis. Review the following risk factors to determine whether you may have an increased chance of developing, or may already have osteoporosis.

Fragility fractures

The occurrence of a fragility fracture, defined as a fracture associated with minimal trauma, virtually proves the presence of osteoporosis. A fragility fracture not only points to the diagnosis, but generally dictates a need for vigorous treatment.

Loss of height of 2 cm or more

Vertebral compression fractures may be associated with significant loss of height. In the person who has been having his or her height measured regularly and accurately, an unexpected decrease in height of even 2 cm may be an important clue. Some loss of height is a normal accompaniment of aging, mainly due to thinning of the intervertebral discs rather than changes in the height of vertebrae. A loss of height of 6cm or more virtually clinches the diagnosis of osteoporosis with vertebral compression fractures.

The development of a stoop or hump in the spine

The development of a stoop and/or a so-called "dowager's hump" in the upper back is likely indicative of vertebral compression fractures and osteoporosis, but it is a late sign.

Female, age 50 or over

Females age 50 or more are at an increased risk for osteoporosis

Past use of glucocorticoid drugs

Significant past use of glucocorticoid drugs, which are used for a variety of immune and inflammatory diseases, is a clear risk factor for osteoporosis and fractures, and should be regarded as an indication to screen for osteoporosis. The National Osteoporosis Foundation of the US has suggested that glucocorticoids in a daily dose equal to or greater than 5 mg per day for three months or longer is an indication for BMD testing.

A positive family history of osteoporosis

A fragility fracture in a first degree relative (parent or sibling) significantly increases the risk of osteoporosis.

Early natural menopause (younger than 45 years) or surgical removal of the ovaries before menopause

Removal of the ovaries for any of a number of reasons will induce an immediate menopause and the associated bone changes, creating the conditions for osteoporosis. This is also the case if the ovaries are not removed but are damaged from radiation treatments or chemotherapy.

Past history of anorexia nervosa

Patients with a history of anorexia nervosa are at increased risk for osteoporosis when they become older, due to effects on their skeleton incurred during periods of reduced food and mineral intake, often associated with cessation of menstruation and estrogen deficiency.

Low body weight (less than 125 lbs or 57 kg) or low body mass index (less than 18.5 kg/m²)

A body weight of less than 125 lbs or 57 kg or a BMI less than 18.5 increases the risk for osteoporosis.

Other lifestyle factors

Moderate or heavy alcohol consumption (three or more drinks per day) increases the risk for osteoporosis. Lifelong low calcium and or vitamin D intake and current smoking also increase risk.

If you have any of these risk factors for osteoporosis, be sure to seek advice from your physician about whether you should have osteoporosis testing.

CHAPTER TWENTY-NINE

What can I do to ensure that I receive a timely diagnosis?

Be proactive

JUST BY READING THIS BOOK, and reviewing your risk factors for osteoporosis, you will be in a position to discuss with your physician, in an informed way, whether you may have osteoporosis, and if so, what action should be taken.

Understand the risk factors for osteoporosis

Review the risk factors for osteoporosis listed in Chapter 28. Determine whether any apply to you and put together whatever information you may have about your past health that may relate to those risk factors.

Be aware of recommendations for bone mineral density assessment, such as those of Osteoporosis Canada

Osteoporosis Canada recommends a bone mineral density measurement for all at age 65, and *earlier if indicated by the presence of risk factors* noted in Chapter 28. Where bone mineral density is not routinely measured at age 65, periodic fracture risk assessment every few years should help to identify individuals who are candidates for bone mineral density measurement, and possibly for active treatment.

Osteoporosis Canada's current recommendations for who should have a bone mineral density measurement are set out in Table 1, Chapter 11. Keep in mind that further development of the FRAX® tool may lead to changes in these recommendations.

Arrange a discussion about osteoporosis with your physician—ask whether you should have a bone mineral density test (DXA)

If you have any of the listed risk factors you have ample reason to discuss with your physician whether you should have a DXA study now, or at some appropriate time in the future. Data are not always available on whether the presence of one or more of these factors should mandate a DXA study—it is a matter of judgment for the patient and his/her physician. Whether or not to do a DXA study should depend on what action would be taken if the bone mineral density value is below normal. A case in point is the pre-menopausal woman (see Chapter 26) in whom drug treatment is unlikely to be started unless the bone mineral density is substantially reduced.

Of course routine bone mineral density measurements on all women at (say) age 55 would at least ensure that the diagnosis is not delayed beyond that age, but for a variety of reasons, including cost, (and, as discussed in Chapter 11, the fact that DXA alone is not a particularly good predictor of who will suffer a fracture in the future) such routine bone mineral density measurements are not being done.

Understand how the FRAX® calculator for fracture risk assessment might help determine whether you should have a bone mineral density assessment

The recently published FRAX® tool (see Chapter 11) calculates the 10-year risk of hip fracture, or of any osteoporotic fracture, based on the patient's values for all proven independent clinical risk factors, with or without a bone mineral density measurement. Once physicians develop experience in using this tool, and more data accumulate, it is likely that it will become an important way of determining who should have a bone mineral density measurement, and for guiding treatment. Not all physicians are using the

FRAX® calculator yet, but it is increasingly becoming part of the osteoporosis assessment process.

Review the bone mineral density report with your physician

Tell your doctor that you would like to understand your bone mineral density results. Review your report with your physician and ask for a copy for your personal records. Increasingly, results are being expressed in terms of absolute fracture risk, rather than a simple T-score or a reference to osteopenia or osteoporosis. Your estimated fracture risk will be one of the factors that determines whether active drug therapy, such as a bisphosphonate, should be started immediately, or whether attention to lifestyle measures is likely to be sufficient, pending a follow-up bone mineral density measurement in two or more years' time.

As noted earlier, the National Osteoporosis Foundation of the US has recommended that the following patients should be considered for treatment. Those with:

- A hip or vertebral fracture, not attributable to major trauma;
- A T-score equal to or less than –2.5 at femoral neck or spine, after excluding secondary causes; or
- A (low) T-score between –1.0 and –2.5 and a 10-year probability of hip fracture equal to or greater than 3% or a probability of a major osteoporosis-related fracture equal to or greater than 20% based on the US-adapted FRAX® calculator.

It should be emphasized that these are guidelines, not a prescription, and each patient needs to be considered on an individual basis, and their preferences taken into account.

If there is no indication for bone mineral density measurement or if it is normal

If there is no indication for a DXA, or if bone mineral density is clearly normal, it is nevertheless prudent to follow the lifestyle measures for osteoporosis prevention discussed in Chapter 16, ensuring an appropriate dietary intake of calcium and vitamin D as well as following an adequate exercise program.

Your osteoporosis physician should provide you with advice on lifestyle, particularly adequate calcium and vitamin D intake and exercise, as well as avoidance of smoking and excess alcohol. In view of the recent concerns regarding calcium supplements and vascular events, large single daily doses of calcium supplements should probably be avoided, especially in older women on no other active treatment. Consideration should also be given to any history of falls, and to any disorders or medications that might increase the risk of falls. Patients should be given specific advice on whether particular activities should be avoided, such as lifting, skiing, hiking over rough terrain and other specific types of exercise, etc.

A decision to follow the lifestyle approach should be accompanied with advice as to when a DXA study might reasonably be expected or repeated. In more borderline cases, a decision might be made to repeat the DXA in two or more years, and at that time, if bone mineral density has declined significantly, the introduction of active drug treatment would need to be considered more seriously.

If a bone mineral density has not yet been done, the patient should be advised whether it is necessary. If a bone mineral density has been done but is normal, there should be agreement whether and when the bone mineral density should be repeated. Unless new risk factors emerge, or a fragility fracture occurs, bone mineral density is usually not repeated in less than two years, in part because the likelihood of a significant change after a shorter time period is very low. Some provincial health programs will not cover the cost of repeat bone mineral density measurements done after an interval of less than two years.

If the bone mineral density is low

If your bone mineral density is low, your physician may wish to do additional tests to rule out secondary osteoporosis, for example due to parathyroid disease. Risk factors should be reviewed and eliminated or reduced wherever possible. If there is any reason to question the adequacy of your vitamin D intake, your physician may order a blood test in order to measure the 25(OH)D level.

If you have a high fracture risk or have had a fragility fracture

In this case, you will certainly require one of the treatments considered in detail in Section 6 of this book. The choice of treatment needs to take many factors into account, including the urgency and severity of the problem, the effectiveness of available treatments, their side-effect profiles, convenience, cost, likelihood of patient adherence, etc. Local considerations including whether certain medications are available in your area and whether they are affordable will need to be taken into account.

At this time, one of the oral bisphosphonates is usually the first-line treatment, but the very encouraging recent experience with infrequent (yearly) intravenous infusions of a bisphosphonate (zoledronate) may herald a changing approach. As we have seen, there is a choice of oral bisphosphonates which can be taken daily, weekly, monthly, or every three months. There may be particular reasons to consider one of the several alternatives to bisphosphonates, including PTH or teriparatide (Forteo), a SERM such as raloxifene, calcitonin, or in the future, strontium ranelate, Denosumab, a SERM other than raloxifene (Evista), or other new treatments.

Once the choice of treatment has been made, it will generally be continued for a prolonged period, measured in years, provided troublesome side-effects do not occur. The most common side-effects from oral bisphosphonates are upper gastro-intestinal symptoms, which the patient may find intolerable. Possible approaches to this problem include switching to an injectable bisphosphonate, or changing to an alternative such as PTH or a SERM.

PTH or teriparatide (Forteo) (by daily subcutaneous injection) will generally be the first choice only under special circumstances, such as very severe osteoporosis or recurrent fractures, in part because it is very expensive. However, the indications may broaden in the future, particularly as the cost falls, or less expensive substitutes are developed. At present, PTH or teriparatide (Forteo) is approved for a maximum course of 18 months in Canada, and it needs to be followed by a course of a bisphosphonate.

CHAPTER THIRTY

Dealing with treatment, monitoring progress and follow-up

Understand the risks versus benefits of treatment

IN DECIDING WHETHER TO START TREATMENT such as a bisphosphonate, it is essential to balance the benefits and the possible risks. Those responsible for marketing drugs may be tempted to emphasize data that show "significant" positive effects, whereas the prescribing physician and the patient should be more interested in whether any benefits are large enough to be clinically meaningful and to outweigh possible side-effects.

Whether or not to treat with drugs may be an easy decision to make in some patient situations and a difficult one in others. For example, it is easy to conclude that a patient with fragility fractures and a low bone mineral density needs active drug treatment. In such a case, it is certainly reasonable for the patient to accept the possibility of side-effects in order to achieve the gains that the medications should provide. It is much less likely that a patient with only a below average bone mineral density, or osteopenia, and with a low fracture risk, will actually benefit from active drug treatment.

As noted in Chapter 29, one of the oral bisphosphonates is usually the first-line treatment. There is a choice of oral bisphosphonates which can be taken daily, weekly, monthly, every three months. There may be particular reasons to consider one of the several alternatives to bisphosphonates, including teriparatide

(Forteo) or PTH, raloxifene (Evista), calcitonin, or in the future, strontium ranelate, Denosumab or other new treatments.

Use of bone mineral density testing (BMD) for monitoring progress

Bone mineral density measurements, using DPX, are widely used for monitoring the progress and treatment of osteoporosis in individual patients. Unfortunately there are misconceptions in the minds of some patients and some physicians regarding the usefulness of such data.

Some of these misconceptions relate to the precision and reproducibility of DPX measurements. Like any other measurement in medicine, the bone mineral density is not 100% precise—if the same patient is measured on different scanners, or if repeat scans are performed on the same scanner, there will be some variation between the results. Factors that may contribute to this include the positioning of the patient on the table (particularly rotation of the hip), and the care and frequency with which the instrument is calibrated.

Each unit should establish its own "least significant change", that is, the magnitude of change in measured bone mineral density which must be observed to be sure that it is a real change. If the least significant change is 4%, that means that any change of less than 4% between successive tests on a given patient is not significant, and cannot be relied upon to guide treatment. A failure to understand this point causes patients and physicians unnecessary concern. If, for example, a patient has been placed on active treatment and shows no increase in bone mineral density after one to two years, or even a 1 or 2% decrease, that does not provide certain proof that the patient is failing to respond.

This is part of the reason why it is futile to repeat DXA measurements too often—it is better to allow an interval during which a change greater than the least significant change can be expected to occur. This often translates into a two year or longer interval rather than a one year interval between bone mineral density measurements.

It is highly desirable that repeat bone mineral density measurements be made on the same machine by an experienced technician. In such circumstances the least significant change will be minimized, and the chance of detecting a significant change correspondingly maximized.

A problem may arise if, between bone mineral density tests, there has been a vertebral compression fracture. This can affect the bone mineral density result and make it less accurate unless the fracture is recognized and taken into account. Fortunately, most bone densitometers now include software which provides an image of the spine, and so any change in the vertebral fracture status from previous tests should be caught by these newer machines. As noted above, in calculating the averaged bone mineral density for the lumbar spine, any vertebrae with evidence of old or recent compression fractures should be excluded from the calculation of the average.

Readers may be wondering how bone mineral density can provide convincing proof that a study drug has caused a 3% increase in bone mineral density after one year, when this is a change that may be less than the least significant change for DXA. The answer, of course, lies in the large number of patients enrolled in such studies. It is the average for the group (those treated versus those not treated) that is being compared, not the individuals' values. If the average gain in bone mineral density over one year in 500 patients (compared with untreated subjects taking a placebo instead of the trial drug) is even 1%, that would be a highly significant increase. If the drug was having no effect, the average change for the 500 patients would be the same as that of the control subjects. This is why large groups of patients are required when we study new drugs. It is only with large groups of subjects that we can identify what may be small but very important results.

It is well recognized that bone mineral density is not the sole determinant of bone strength. It is influenced by the remodeling rate. Defects in the protein (collagen) or in the bone mineral (apatite) of the bone, or microstructural abnormalities such as microfractures may also affect bone strength.

An important observation that has emerged from clinical trials of many of the new active treatments for osteoporosis is that the improvement in fracture risk does not necessarily parallel changes in bone mineral density. In many of the studies, a marked reduction in fractures has been observed before the bone mineral density has changed significantly. Presumably the treatment is strengthening the bone through changes independent of bone mineral density, such as a decrease in the bone remodeling rate, which may become apparent within weeks of starting treatment.

Keep with your program and make sure you get good follow-up

The patient (as well as the physician) should ensure that, as far as possible, repeat bone mineral density determinations are performed on the same machine to maximize the chances of detecting significant changes.

Adherence to recommended treatment is a major problem in osteoporosis management. This is not a problem that is peculiar to osteoporosis, but rather it is a very common problem in chronic medical disorders, particularly those in which there are few symptoms.

We have discussed some of the issues with calcium supplements (see Chapter 16). In some patients, increasing the intake of dairy products may be more acceptable, and better adhered to, than calcium supplements in pill or liquid form. It is also possible that calcium ingested in the food might not share with calcium supplements any tendency to increase vascular events (if that is confirmed to be a genuine concern), though this would need to be proved. Adherence to vitamin D supplements should be less of a problem in the future if occasional large doses replace the present more frequent dosing.

Continuation with an exercise program may be one of the more important things a patient can do to help themself. Both the patient and those caring for her/him should do everything possible to minimize the risk of falls.

Taking your medication regularly and continuously is very important

It is important to understand that drug treatment carries on for years, not weeks or months. You must be sure to keep going with the treatment as long as your physician recommends it in order to achieve the benefits of the medication. Not everyone seems able to do this and this has had an important impact on the outcome of osteoporosis treatment. In the case of bisphosphonates, for example, adherence to the usual once weekly regime with alendronate (Fosamax) and risedronate (Actonel) is surprisingly poor, as determined by checking whether pills have been dispensed, and by counting the pills remaining at the end of a prescribed period. Average adherence may be as low as 50%, and no doubt it is much lower in some patients. Although symptoms (usually gastrointestinal) and cost may contribute to non-adherence, they do not appear to be the primary cause. More often it reflects the disinclination of patients to take a medication regularly for a condition presently causing few or no symptoms. This is an area where patient education and the patient's cooperation in the planned treatment can make a very real difference. It is obviously essential that patients are honest with their physician regarding adherence to medications, otherwise it is not possible to manage the osteoporosis satisfactorily.

Likewise, getting the requested investigations done (particularly follow-up bone mineral densities where these are indicated), and attending follow-up appointments is a necessary part of the care program. Bone mineral density will generally be repeated after at least two, and, rarely one years of treatment. Decisions regarding continued treatment will be based on clinical considerations (e.g. absence of further fractures) as well as the bone mineral density.

It has already been emphasized that fracture prevention does not closely parallel the change in bone mineral density, so the treatment regimen need not necessarily be changed just because the patient's bone mineral density has not shown significant improvement. In the future other techniques which give information on bone quality as well as quantity, such as micro-CT, may be used to provide more comprehensive information on treatment response, and may be particularly helpful in patients who do not appear to be responding satisfactorily to treatment. Bone markers can be measured under special circumstances, for example to confirm that bone resorption is appropriately suppressed in the patient on a bisphosphonate.

If treatment is having the desired effect, bone mineral density testing may not be needed as frequently as every two years in every patient. It is important to remember that an unchanged bone mineral density may be an entirely satisfactory response, especially where it was previously declining. Questions remain as to how long treatment should carry on. Early research data suggests that, provided the patient is not fracturing and the bone mineral density is not very low, bisphosphonates may be discontinued after five years in some patients.

If treatment is failing

If treatment is clearly failing, the first steps should be to ensure that lifestyle measures are being followed properly, that medications are being taken correctly and regularly, and that there are no secondary causes for the osteoporosis. If no explanation for the poor response is identified, a change is indicated, usually to a drug with a different mode of action from that which has failed, for example from bisphosphonate to teriparatide (Forteo) or PTH or (when it becomes available) to strontium ranelate. Here again, bone markers might be useful in guiding treatment towards an anabolic rather than an antiresorptive drug, or vice-versa (see Chapter 7).

What can I expect from my osteoporosis physician?

It will be apparent to readers of this guide that there are a number of issues, even in the uncomplicated patient, where choices have to be made, and complete data are not necessarily available to make a scientific decision. Furthermore, advances are continually being made, and the patient needs to be provided with up-to-date information as well as advice on how to interpret it.

There will be plenty of issues you will want to discuss, including:

1. Do I really have an important increase in my risk of fracturing, as opposed to a below-average bone mineral density that is not clinically significant?
2. Have secondary causes of osteoporosis been adequately excluded?
3. Are lifestyle measures sufficient, with a follow-up bone mineral density measurement some time in the future, to determine if additional drug treatment needs to be added, or should drug therapy begin immediately?
4. If drug therapy is required immediately, which drug should be given (e.g. bisphosphonate, raloxifene (Evista), teriparatide (Forteo) (PTH), or strontium ranelate when available, etc?)
5. Assuming the medication is tolerated, what follow-up should be planned and in particular, should the bone mineral density be repeated, and if so, when?
6. How do we judge whether a change in measured bone mineral density is meaningful?
7. Assuming clinical and bone mineral density response is satisfactory, how long should the drug be continued? This is a particular issue with bisphosphonates.
8. If clinical or bone mineral density response is not satisfactory, should a change of drug therapy be considered, and if so, when?

Maintain a positive attitude

As with all chronic medical ailments, the importance of the patient's attitude cannot be over stated. As physicians, we have all seen individuals severely affected by osteoporosis with a positive attitude to life, who manage to remain active, in contrast to others who allow themselves to become severely disabled in the face of apparently much milder disease. The use of the unfortunate term "osteopenia" has engendered a lot of unnecessary anxiety, sometimes leading patients to believe that they have a 'disease' when, in fact, their bone mineral density is merely below average. The physician should be able to foster more positive attitudes by dispelling such misconceptions, and by pointing out that the outlook in osteoporosis is much better than it was a few decades ago, and that there are now a variety of effective treatments for the disorder.

Keep informed on progress in osteoporosis

We do not yet have answers to many important questions regarding the management of osteoporosis, so for the foreseeable future, as with many chronic disorders, the patient will need to rely on the judgment of their osteoporosis physician, together with any reliable information they can glean from other sources. As physicians treating osteoporosis, we welcome the accessibility of reliable, accurate information on the internet as well as in print, so that interested patients can find out more about what is available. It is refreshing, although sometimes challenging, to encounter a patient in the clinic setting who is knowledgeable about the options, and can ask appropriate questions. Unfortunately evidence-based answers to these questions may not be available, and only continuing research will provide the physician and the patient with the answers we both seek.

PART FOUR | **Special topics**

Special topics in osteoporosis

CHAPTER THIRTY-ONE

Glucocorticoid-induced osteoporosis

Glucocorticoids

GLUCOCORTICOIDS ARE RELATED to the naturally occurring hormone, cortisol, which is produced by the adrenal glands. Doctors usually refer to these drugs as "steroids" but they are not the same steroids that are used by some athletes, which are related to testosterone. Prednisone is the most widely used glucocorticoid. Glucocorticoids are very effective anti-inflammatory agents and also suppress the immune system. They have been in use for many years to treat a wide range of inflammatory and immune diseases, including rheumatoid arthritis, asthma and transplants.

Long-term glucocorticoid use can lead to side-effects in virtually every organ in the body, including muscles and bones. Osteoporosis and fractures may occur, as well as muscle weakness. The severity of these side-effects is related to the dose and duration of glucocorticoid treatment. The bone loss caused by glucocorticoid use is most rapid in the first 12–18 months, and then continues at a slower rate. Glucocorticoids are the most common cause of secondary osteoporosis.

How is osteoporosis caused by glucocorticoids?

There appear to be several mechanisms, of which the most important is decreased osteoblast activity and therefore decreased bone formation. Glucocorticoids reduce collagen formation by osteoblasts and reduce osteoblast life span. They increase osteocyte apoptosis, which may adversely affect the maintenance of bone quality. There is an early increase in osteoclast activity and prolongation of osteoclast life span. All of these effects decrease bone mass. Perhaps as a result of decreased osteoblast numbers, the microarchitecture of trabeculae deteriorates, with thinning and perforation, further weakening the bone. Glucocorticoids also decrease the absorption of calcium by the intestine, and this, together with increases in urinary calcium losses, may contribute to an increase in PTH.

A separate and serious disorder of bone associated with glucocorticoids is called "avascular necrosis" (avascular means lacking blood supply). In this disorder, there is local necrosis (death) of areas of bone, usually near the hip, shoulder and knee joints, causing pain and sometimes requiring joint replacement. The mechanism through which glucocorticoids cause avascular necrosis is not fully understood, but a reduction in the number of osteocytes (as a result of apoptosis) may interfere with bone health. The effect of glucocorticoids on muscle, leading to weakness and decreased mobility, may also contribute to bone loss, weakness, instability and fractures.

How common is glucocorticoid-induced osteoporosis?

It has been estimated that osteoporosis occurs in up to 50% of patients on long-term glucocorticoids. Vertebral fractures are particularly frequent in postmenopausal women receiving glucocorticoids, occurring in up to 20% of patients in the first year, presumably depending on the bone mineral density before glucocorticoid treatment and the underlying condition for which the glucocorticoids were given. The dose and duration of glucocorticoid treatment are important, but significant bone loss can occur even with as low a dose as 5 mg of prednisone or equivalent for three months or longer. Inhaled glucocorticoids have less effect on bone than glucocorticoids given by mouth, but they can contribute to the development of osteoporosis, depending on the inhaled dose.

Investigations

Bone loss from glucocorticoids is greatest from trabecular bone, so it can be detected early with a CT bone mineral density study of the spine. However, this is not generally available, and requires a higher radiation dose than DXA, so DXA is more commonly used. There is some evidence that fractures occur at higher bone mineral densities in glucocorticoid-induced osteoporosis than in other types of osteoporosis. This suggests that interventions might be appropriate at a higher bone mineral density (higher than –2.5) in glucocorticoid-induced osteoporosis.

A baseline bone mineral density should be done in patients who are starting on what is expected to be long-term glucocorticoid treatment. Since losses of 5–10% per year may occur from the spine, bone mineral density measurements should be done more frequently than in the usual osteoporosis patient—for example every 12 months. Glucocorticoid bone loss may be reversible on stopping glucocorticoid treatment. Biochemical bone markers (see Chapter 7) show an abrupt decline in bone formation on starting glucocorticoids. However, these are not useful in managing the clinical problem and so they are not routinely measured.

Prevention and treatment of glucocorticoid-induced osteoporosis

Doses of glucocorticoids should be kept to a minimum, and the usual attention should be given to lifestyle issues—adequate calcium and vitamin D intake, exercise and avoidance of falls, and reduction or cessation of smoking and excessive alcohol intake.

Hormone replacement

There is some evidence that bone mineral density is improved by estrogen in women, and by testosterone in men, who are taking glucocorticoids. However, more effective treatments than hormone replacement are available.

Calcium and vitamin D

Calcium supplements alone have been shown not to be sufficient to prevent bone loss due to glucocorticoid treatment. Calcium plus vitamin D appears to be more effective. Some studies have suggested that the active form of vitamin D normally produced in the kidneys ($1,25(OH)_2D$) may be more effective than regular vitamin D for preventing glucocorticoid-induced bone loss. One alphahydroxy D, which is converted to $1,25(OH)_2D$ in the body, has also been used, but was shown to be less effective than alendronate (Fosamax) for glucocorticoid-induced osteoporosis.

Calcitonin and bisphosphonates

Calcitonin has been shown to reduce glucocorticoid-induced bone loss in some studies, but not in others. There have been numerous studies of bisphosphonates in prevention and treatment of glucocorticoid-induced osteoporosis. Several studies have demonstrated their effectiveness. Didronel significantly decreased bone loss. Alendronate (Fosamax) with calcium and vitamin D caused an increase in bone mineral density in patients recently started on glucocorticoids, whereas in the patients on calcium and vitamin D alone, there was significant bone loss. Similarly, risedronate (Actonel) prevented bone loss, and there was a suggestion of a reduction in vertebral fractures with both drugs.

Parathyroid hormone and teriparatide (Forteo)

Teriparatide (Forteo) or PTH would be predicted to be effective in glucocorticoid-induced osteoporosis, which mainly results from reduced osteoblastic activity. In a study in postmenopausal women with glucocorticoid-induced osteoporosis, PTH plus estrogens increased lumbar spine bone mineral density (by DXA) by 11% in one year, whereas there was no change in the group given estrogens alone. A recent study in women and men with glucocorticoid-induced osteoporosis directly compared teriparatide (Forteo) with oral alendronate (Fosamax) in usual doses for 18 months. Teriparatide (Forteo) produced a significantly greater increase in bone mineral density than alendronate (Fosamax) at both spine and hip, and was also associated with fewer new vertebral (but not non-vertebral) fractures.

Summary

Any patient requiring 5 mg per day or more of prednisone (or equivalent), for three months or more, with a T-score less than

–2.5 or a high fracture risk, should receive oral or intravenous bisphosphonate, or teriparatide (Forteo). Both bisphosphonates and teriparatide (Forteo) are effective for the prevention and treatment of glucocorticoid-induced osteoporosis. The choice between these agents will depend in part on the relative costs and on whether specific contraindications are present to the use of either group of agents. Particularly in postmenopausal women, active treatment should be considered if the T-score is less than –1.5. If bisphosphonate is not indicated, calcium and vitamin D is recommended, with annual follow-up and perhaps annual bone mineral density measurement to review whether more active treatment may be indicated.

CHAPTER THIRTY-TWO

Osteoporosis in the transplant patient

TRANSPLANTATION OF THE KIDNEY, liver, heart, lung and bone marrow are now accepted treatments. Many of the diseases that lead to failure of the respective organ that needs to be replaced can themselves affect bone. Furthermore, several of the drugs used in managing the transplant patient, particularly those used to prevent or treat rejection of the transplant, including glucocorticoids, also affect bone.

Because glucocorticoids suppress the immune system, they were originally the mainstay for the prevention of transplant rejection, and were used in large doses for long periods of time. The significant effects of glucocorticoids on bone are discussed in Chapter 31. Glucocorticoids are still used in patients with transplants, but the introduction of a number of effective new anti-rejection drugs, such as azathioprine (Imuran) and more recently cyclosporine and tacrolimus has made possible the use of lower doses of glucocorticoids. Hopefully this will result in fewer bone issues amongst transplant patients.

Cyclosporine and tacrolimus

The direct effects of these drugs on human bone are not clear. By allowing for the use of less glucocorticoids, they may reduce glucocorticoid damage to the skeleton.

Kidney transplant

Kidney transplant patients often have pre-existing bone disease related to kidney failure. In addition, there is rapid loss of bone mineral density immediately after transplantation. Fractures of peripheral bones (hips and limbs) are more common than fractures of vertebrae.

Heart and liver transplant

Early loss of bone mineral density occurs in heart and liver transplant patients. Fractures of vertebrae are particularly frequent.

Prevention and treatment of transplant osteoporosis

It has been suggested that patients awaiting heart, liver and lung transplantation should have a skeletal evaluation, and be considered for bisphosphonate treatment before transplant. It is hoped that this will decrease post-transplant bone loss. Fewer data are available for patients awaiting kidney transplant in whom bisphosphonates are generally not safe for use because of their low level of kidney function.

In the early post-transplant period, vitamin D, particularly $1,25(OH)_2D$, may help to preserve bone mass.

Bisphosphonates are currently the treatment of choice for the prevention and treatment of transplant osteoporosis. Intravenous bisphosphonates (ibandronate (Boniva) and zoledronic acid (Aclasta)) have a significant protective effect on bone mass, and may be more effective than bisphosphonates taken by mouth. However, intravenous bisphosphonates have the potential to cause kidney damage, and this may limit their use. The optimal duration of treatment has not been determined, and there is concern about the possibility of "frozen bone" in kidney transplant patients (see Chapter 19).

Hormone replacement is recommended in young (premenopausal) women who develop cessation of menstruation (amenorrhea) after transplant, as they will otherwise be exposed to the bone effects that are seen in postmenopausal women.

APPENDICES

Appendix I: *Control of osteoclasts*

Appendix II: *Control of osteoblasts*

Appendix III: **DXA Bone Density Report**

Appendix IV: **Calcium intake calculator**

Appendix I: Control of osteoclasts

OSTEOCLASTS ARE FORMED by the fusion of several macrophages, which are a type of cell found in the bone marrow. The process of osteoclast formation is triggered by a reaction between two proteins – one on the surface of macrophages, called RANK, and the other on osteoclasts, called RANKL. Another protein, osteoprotegerin, interferes with this interaction, and in a strain of mice in which osteoprotegerin is present in excess, too few osteoclasts are formed and consequently the bones are abnormally dense.

A similar end result—abnormally dense bones due to too few osteoclasts—results from a rare mutation of the RANKL gene in humans. A human monoclonal antibody that binds to RANKL has been developed commercially, and is known as Denosumab. It decreases the interaction of RANK and RANKL, therefore decreasing osteoclasts, and has been shown in clinical trials to increase BMD and reduce fractures in postmenopausal women when given by subcutaneous injection (see Denosumab treatment). Another piece of evidence indicating the importance of RANKL and osteoprotegerin in humans is the recent discovery that regions of the genome close to each of these genes are linked with bone mineral density.

Osteoclasts remove bone by creating a space between osteoclast and bone surface which can be made very acidic (and hence dissolve bone mineral) and into which are secreted enzymes that dissolve the bone matrix. One of these enzymes is Cathepsin K. An inherited lack of Cathepsin K is associated with abnormally dense bones. Odanacatib is a new drug that inhibits the action of Cathepsin K and is currently undergoing trials as a potential treatment for osteoporosis. Odanacatib has an entirely different mode of action from all other treatments and is an exciting new area of osteoporosis research.

Appendix II: Control of osteoblasts

VERY RECENT RESEARCH HAS SUGGESTED that there is a link between the development of osteoblasts and that of fat cells. Both of these cell types appear to be derived from the same parent cell in the bone marrow. Factors that increase the production of fat may, at the same time, decrease the formation of osteoblasts and therefore contribute to osteoporosis. For example, studies in animals have shown that rosiglitazone (an antidiabetic drug that has been associated with an may divert stem cells towards becoming fat cells rather than osteoblasts.

Many proteins are involved in the formation and activation of osteoblasts, including insulin-like growth factor (IGF-1), sclerostin and others. Sclerostin is thought to be involved in signaling between osteocytes and the bone remodeling units. Inactivation of the sclerostin gene in humans causes increased osteoblast activity and disorders with increased bone density, including a condition called sclerosteosis, which may be associated with some bone deformities. Antibodies against sclerostin have been shown to increase bone mass in experimental animals, and are already undergoing early clinical trials in human osteoporosis.

PTH may exert its anabolic effect in osteoporosis in part by decreasing sclerostin, allowing greater stimulation of osteoblastic activity. However, the ability of PTH to cause increased bone removal under some circumstances, and bone formation under others, is still incompletely understood. With prolonged PTH administration by daily subcutaneous injection to humans, bone markers show that increased bone formation occurs early, but after a year or more, bone resorption (removal) predominates. This has been described as the "anabolic window"—the time when the beneficial effect of PTH on bone mineral density may be most likely to occur.

Growth hormone, produced by the pituitary gland, works partly by increasing IGF-1 production by the liver. Growth hormone and IGF-1 increase bone mineral density when given to treat individuals with deficiencies of these hormones, which are usually associated with growth retardation. IGF-1 is also deficient in anorexia nervosa, and it is being explored as a possible treatment for osteoporosis associated with anorexia nervosa. Insufficient research has been done to show whether growth hormone or IGF-1 have a place in the treatment of osteoporosis that is not associated with deficiency of these hormones.

Appendix III: DXA Bone Density Report

Female T- and Z-scores for lumbar vertebrae (L1-L4)

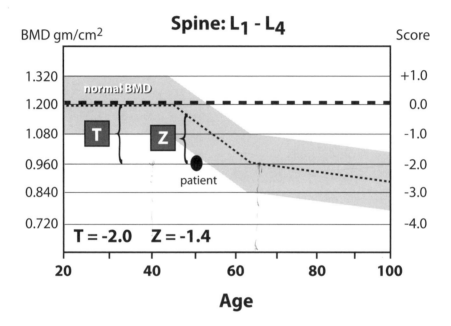

THE BONE MINERAL DENSITY (BMD) is shown as grams of mineral per square centimeter scanned (gm/cm2) on the left, and standard deviation (SD) score on the right of the figure. The horizontal (heavy, dashed) zero line is the average BMD value for a normal young adult female. The grey band shows the normal BMD, plus or minus one standard deviation in normal females, with the average value shown as the dotted line in the middle of the grey band. BMD falls rapidly around the time of menopause, between ages 40 and 60, and more slowly in post-menopausal women.

T-scores compare the patient's BMD with that of a young normal adult—the zero line in the figure. The difference between the patient's score and the zero line is expressed as the number of SDs; one SD usually equals 10 to 15% of the BMD value in gm/cm2.

Z-scores compare the patient's BMD with the expected average BMD for the patient's age and sex—the dotted line in the figure, and again the difference is expressed as the number of SDs.

The example shown in the figure as "patient" is a 50 year-old woman with a BMD of 0.960 gm/cm². As explained in chapters 8 and 26, the T-score is used for reporting the BMD in post-menopausal women. Hence, if this is a 50-year-old post-menopausal woman, the BMD would be reported as a T-score of –2.0, which would place her in the "osteopenia" range (between –1.0 and –2.5). If this 50-year-old woman were still pre-menopausal, her BMD would be reported as the Z-score of –1.4, which is normal. As discussed in chapter 26, Z-scores below –2.0 in pre-menopausal women are described as "low bone mineral density", and the terms osteopenia and osteoporosis are not generally used.

Note that a BMD of 0.960 gm/cm² represents a T-score of –2.0 at any age, whereas the Z-score corresponding to a BMD of 0.960 gm/cm² is dependent upon the patient's age. Reference to the figure shows that at age 40 the Z-score corresponding to a BMD of 0.960 gm/cm² is –2.0, whereas at age 65 the corresponding Z-score for this BMD is 0.0.

Appendix IV: Calcium Intake Calculator

(BC Dairy Foundation)

Approx. calcium content per portion	Foods	Portion size	Number of portions	Total portions	x mg per portion	Total milligrams of calcium
	Milk – skim, 1%, 2%, whole buttermilk or chocolate	1 cup	_____			
	Calcium fortified beverages (ie soy, rice)	1 cup	_____			**A**
	Skim milk powder	$1/3$ cup	_____			
300 mg	Yogurt, plain (reg or low fat)	$3/4$ cup	_____	_____	x 300 =	☐ mg
	Firm cheese such as cheddar, swiss, gouda, reg or low fat	$11/4$ cube	_____			
	Processed cheese slices (reg or low fat)	2 slices	_____			**B**
	Salmon canned, with bones or Sardines canned, with bones	$1/2$ can	_____			
250 mg	Yogurt, fruit-flavored reg or low fat	$3/4$ cup	_____	_____	x 250 =	☐ mg
	Baked, soy or white beans	1 cup	_____			
	Ice milk, frozen yogurt (reg or low fat)	$1/2$ cup	_____			
	Pancakes or waffles made with milk	3 medium	_____			
	Pudding	$1/2$ cup	_____			
	Soy, semi-soft cheese (feta, mozza, camembert reg or low fat)	$11/4$ cube	_____			**C**
	Soup made with milk	1 cup	_____			
150 mg	Tofu made with calcium	3 oz	_____	_____	x 150 =	☐ mg
	Bok choy or kale, cooked	$1/2$ cup	_____			
	Chickpeas	1 cup	_____			
	Cottage cheese (reg or low fat)	$1/2$ cup	_____			
	Ice cream	$1/2$ cup	_____			**D**
	Parmesan cheese	1 Tbsp	_____			
75 mg	Almonds	$1/4$ cup	_____	_____	x 75 =	☐ mg
	Bread	2 slices	_____			
	Broccoli	$3/4$ cup	_____			**E**
	Kulver beans, lima beans, lentils	1 cup	_____			
50 mg	Orange (fruit, not juice)	1 medium	_____	_____	x 75 =	☐ mg

Daily Calcium Intake = Sum of A + B + C + D + E = ☐ mg

Glossary

Alkaline phosphatase: An enzyme produced by osteoblasts during bone formation.

Anabolic drugs: Drugs for the treatment of osteoporosis whose main action is to increase osteoblastic new bone formation.

Antiresorptive drugs: Drugs for the treatment of osteoporosis whose main action is to decrease osteoclastic bone removal.

Apatite: The calcium mineral (calcium phosphate) that makes bone hard and is assessed by bone mineral density tests.

Apoptosis: A process of programmed death of cells when their function is completed.

Avascular necrosis: Death of tissues resulting from a loss of their blood supply. Often refers to death of the head of the femur after certain forms of hip fracture.

Biochemical markers: Substances which can be measured in blood or urine samples and are indicators of the rates of bone removal and bone formation occurring in the skeleton.

Bone densitometry: Measurement of bone mineral density.

Bone matrix proteins: The protein component of bone, including collagen, osteocalcin and other proteins.

Bone mineral density: The quantity of bone mineral in an area of bone, usually expressed as calcium per unit quantity of bone.

Bone remodeling (or bone multicellular) units (BRUs): Discrete microscopic regions within trabecular and cortical bone where bone remodeling is occurring.

Bone turnover: The normal process of removal of old bone and replacement by new bone occurring in the skeleton throughout life.

BRU: see Bone remodeling unit.

Calcaneus: The heel bone.

Calcium carbonate: A simple and inexpensive form of calcium supplementation (chalk).

Calcium phosphate: A compound in which calcium and phosphate are bound together.

Calcium sensing receptor (CaSR): The protein receptor on the surface of parathyroid (and other) cells which senses the calcium level in the blood.

Celiac disease: An inflammatory disease of the small intestine resulting from sensitivity to wheat protein (gluten), which leads to poor absorption of some substances from the intestine.

Collagen: A protein forming strong fibers which is present in several body tissues including bone and skin. It is the major non-mineral portion of bone.

Compression fractures: Fractures in which the bone (usually a vertebral body) is squashed (compressed) leading to a loss of height and deformation of the spine.

Cortical bone: Dense bone, usually forming a solid cylinder (as in the shafts of the long bones of the limbs), or surrounding the spongy trabecular bone (as in the vertebral bodies).

CT bone densitometry (QCT): Bone mineral density determined by computerized tomography (CT) usually focused on the trabecular bone of the vertebrae.

Dual photon X-ray absorptiometry test (DXA): The standard test for measuring bone mineral density, most commonly at spine and hip.

Elemental calcium: Pure calcium, or the amount of pure calcium in a compound. For example only 40% of the compound calcium carbonate, one of the most common calcium supplements, is elemental calcium.

Estrogen: Female sex hormone produced in the ovaries.

Family history: The history of disease (commonly genetic) in an individual's family.

Femoral head: The top of the femur (thigh) bone. The femoral head is the ball of the 'ball-and-socket' joint of the hip. It sits atop the femoral neck (see below). Part of the blood supply of the femoral head comes from vessels that travel upward to the head along the femoral neck. In hip fractures that involve the femoral neck, these vessels may be disrupted leading to death of the femoral head from lack of blood supply. In such cases, the femoral head may have to be replaced by an artificial head.

Femoral neck: The short portion of the femur (thigh) bone that lies between the "ball" at the top of the femur and the long shaft of the femur. This is often where hip fractures occur.

Fracture Risk Assessment Tool (FRAX®): A method for estimating fracture risk over 10 years. Developed by the World Heath Organization (WHO). Available online at *www.shef.ac.uk/FRAX*.

Fragility fractures: Fractures that occur from minimal trauma, e.g. after a fall from standing height or less. These are usually a sign of osteoporosis.

Glucocorticoids: Cortisone-related drugs used to treat inflammatory disease. Sometimes known as "steroids."

Hormone replacement therapy: Administration of estrogen and progesterone at or following the time of menopause.

HRpQCT (High resolution peripheral quantitative CT): A high resolution 3-dimensional CT scan of bone, e.g. the wrist.

Hypercalcemia: An abnormally high level of calcium in the blood.

Immature bone: Newly formed bone, not yet fully mineralized.

Kyphoplasty: Inflation of a balloon inside a recently fractured and compressed vertebra to permit injection of cement into the space created after the balloon is removed. This is a minimally invasive surgical procedure, mainly used to relieve pain from compression fractures of the vertebrae.

Kyphosis: Increased spinal curvature leading to prominence of the upper back and a forward "hunch" of the neck and head.

Lining cells: The layer of inactive cells covering the bone surface in areas where remodeling is not occurring.

Macrophages: Cells with the capacity to engulf foreign material.

Mature bone: Older bone in which bone mineral crystallization (apatite) is complete.

Microfractures: Microscopic (tiny) fractures or cracks within trabecular or cortical bone.

Mineralization: Deposition of apatite (calcium phosphate) on a protein (collagen) base or matrix. This is what makes bone hard.

Modeling: The process by which a bone changes shape during growth.

Nafarelin treatment for endometriosis: Nafarelin (synarel) is a medication, usually given by nasal spray, which suppresses the release of the pituitary hormones LH and FSH, which leads to reduced estrogen production by the ovaries. Endometriosis is a disorder of the endometrium (the lining of the womb) which is made worse by the presence of estrogen, and is improved by long-term estrogen suppression. However, long-term estrogen suppression has adverse effects on the bone, promoting the development of osteoporosis.

Osteoarthritis: Degenerative disease of the joints often associated with age or previous injury.

Osteoblasts: The cells responsible for new bone formation in BRUs.

Osteocalcin: A protein unique to bone, produced by osteoblasts during bone formation, and also released into the blood during osteoclastic bone resorption.

Osteoclasts: The cells responsible for bone removal or resorption in BRUs.

Osteocytes: The network of inter-connected cells lying in spaces (lacunae) within mineralized bone. Osteocytes are derived from osteoblasts and function as sensors within the bone.

Osteogenesis imperfecta: A genetic form of osteoporosis usually presenting in a very severe form in early life.

Osteomalacia: Bone disease resulting from severe vitamin D deficiency with a characteristic microscopic appearance that shows a failure to mineralize collagen.

Osteopenia: A reduced level of bone mineralization, not sufficiently reduced to be called osteoporosis.

Osteoporosis: A generalized condition of the skeleton with reduced bone mineral density and deterioration of bone quality, leading to an increased risk of fractures.

Paget's disease: A disorder of bone of unknown cause with a patchy distribution in which osteoclasts are present in excessive numbers, the bone often expands and may be painful.

Parathyroid glands: Four small glands in the neck which control the calcium level in the blood.

Parathyroid hormone (PTH): The hormone produced by the parathyroid glands to regulate the calcium level in the blood.

Peak bone mass: The maximum bone mineral density achieved during an individual's life, which occurs in early adulthood.

Perforations: Gaps in trabeculae due to osteoclastic bone removal. Also called "loss of connectivity."

Porosity: Pores (cavities) in cortical bone resulting from increased bone resorption.

Postmenopausal osteoporosis: Osteoporosis following the female menopause.

Precursor cells: Cells which are the parents of certain special cells such as osteoclasts or osteoblasts.

Primary hyperparathyroidism (PHP): Overactivity of one or more of the parathyroid glands.

Primary mineralization: The first phase of deposition of apatite onto newly formed collagen bone matrix.

Primary osteoporosis: Osteoporosis in the absence of any identifiable underlying cause.

Progesterone: Female sex hormone produced by the ovary following ovulation.

Protein: A substance composed of a sequence of amino acids. The shape and behavior of a protein is determined by the sequence. Proteins are the essential component of all living matter.

Pulmonary embolism: A detached blood clot from a vein that flows in the blood stream through the heart and lodges in the lung(s).

Quantitative ultrasound (QUS): An instrument which uses ultrasound to assess the quality and quantity of bone, commonly in the heel. This test has gained some popularity as a simple, fast and inexpensive way of diagnosing osteoporosis but there is, as yet, only moderate evidence confirming its value.

Resorption cavity: The cavity produced by the action of osteoclasts during bone remodeling.

Remodeling: The normal process of removal of old bone and replacement by new bone which occurs throughout the skeleton and throughout life. Occurs within bone remodeling units (BRUs).

Rickets: Vitamin D deficiency bone disorder of childhood.

Secondary mineralization: The later phase of mineralization during which apatite crystals become larger and more uniform, and bone mineral density increases.

Secondary osteoporosis: Osteoporosis due to (secondary to) an identifiable disease, medication or other causes.

Single photon absorptiometers (SPAs): An early type of bone densitometer for testing bone mineral density, suitable only for bones without much overlying muscle and other tissue—e.g. forearm bones.

Standard deviation: A statistical measure that shows the dispersion of values within a population.

Steroids: see Glucocorticoids.

Stiffness index: A theoretical index of bone stiffness derived from QUS measurements in which an ultrasound beam passes through bone.

Trabeculae: The fine struts and plates within trabecular (spongy) bone.

Trabecular bone: Spongy bone consisting of fine struts and plates (trabeculae) present in the interior of some bones, for example the spinal vertebrae. Often surrounded by denser and harder cortical bone.

Venous thrombosis: Blood clotting in the veins.

Vertebral bodies: The blocks of bone forming the spinal column.

Vertebral fracture assessment (VFA): The X-ray image of the spine provided by modern DXA instruments for the identification of vertebral compression fractures. The quality of the image is not as good as a conventional spine X-ray, but it requires a much lower dose of X-rays, and is adequate for most clinical purposes.

Vertebroplasty: Injection of cement into a recently compressed vertebra, mainly used for the relief of severe pain.

Vitamin D: A fat soluble vitamin involved in the formation and health of bone.

Index